A POLICE SURGEON'S LOT

30 years in the real world of a West Country Police Surgeon

Dr. Peter Moore

"The mood and temper of the public in regard to the treatment of crime and criminals is one of the most unfailing tests of the civilization of any country."

Winston S Churchill

Copyright © 2016 Dr. Peter Moore
All rights reserved.

ISBN: 1530650410
ISBN 13: 9781530650415

This book is dedicated to Detective Inspector Arthur Moore, my brother, close friend and senior police officer who never gave up.

Dr Nick Fisher, a colleague, friend and amazing police surgeon.

Introduction	A night in the cells	vii
Chapter 1	What am I doing here?	1
Chapter 2	Real murder most foul	6
Chapter 3	I cannot face tomorrow	24
Chapter 4	Mad, Bad or Sad	39
Chapter 5	Not like sex at all	57
Chapter 6	I'll drive; I'm too drunk to sing.	79
Chapter 7	Just a scratch	96
Chapter 8	The drug scene	114
Chapter 9	Problems with booze	129
Chapter 10	One for the pot – Cannabis	138
Chapter 11	Downers; From opium to Valium	146
Chapter 12	More haste less speed	158
Chapter 13	Nothing but the truth.	174
Chapter 14	You're nicked son	190
Chapter 15	Anything you say	203
Chapter 16	Born evil?	215
Chapter 17	All change	225
References		239

INTRODUCTION
A NIGHT IN THE CELLS

5th September 2001.

I arrived at Torquay Custody Centre at ten to nine in the evening and parked in the yard, behind the police station. I let myself in with my pass key and Sergeant Mills, the custody sergeant on duty, told me that Michelle Downes was in again. She was well known to the police and the drug addiction services. This was a routine call. I knew that I might be called at any time to see a body or a rape victim.

She looked unkempt and more than her twenty-five years when I saw her in the medical room. She was underweight, with sunken cheeks, wearing old jeans and t shirt. There was no eye contact as she looked down at the desk; did she even know I was there? A female detention officer stayed with me.

"I'm rattling Doc," were her first words. I explained who I was, a doctor independent from the police, and that anything she said would be confidential unless I was ordered to disclose it by a court. I doubt that she understood a word. She normally injected a hundred and forty pounds' worth of heroin every day. She bought it on the streets in ten pound wraps; having no idea how much pure heroin was in each wrap or what else she was injecting into her veins. She was almost certainly hepatitis C positive; in my experience, they all are.

She claimed that her last hit had been at 04-00 am nearly seventeen hours before but I was used to addicts lying. She knew that I would not prescribe a top-up if she admitted that she had been injecting within the previous six hours.

She told me that she also took diazepam, an addictive tranquillizer. She had seen drug addiction workers and had been on lofexidine but had dropped out of the programme. She hardly touched alcohol.

She was born in Manchester and went to a "normal" school. She had even passed some GCSEs and started to study sport science but, at eighteen, had started using heroin. She also had a seven-year-old child who was in care.

She complained of abdominal cramps and generalised aching. Her motions had been loose. These were classic signs of heroin withdrawal but were there any objective signs? I could not rely on anything she told me. If she had been withdrawing from Heroin she should have some of the classic signs; large pupils, a raised blood pressure and pulse, "goosebumps" on the skin, yawning and a runny nose. Objectively everything was normal. Although she was telling me the classic symptoms of heroin withdrawal, this did not fit the results of my physical examination. I had to determine whether she was over-egging the pudding to make me prescribe.

She fully understood the allegations against her, had good recall and knew the set up. This was not going to be her first police interview. I decided that she was fit to be detained and did not need any medication yet.

I then saw a young man, also in his twenties. He came into the medical room at ten past nine, after I had spent twenty minutes with Michelle. Again, I explained my role and the problems regarding confidentiality. Again, I doubted that he understood.

He was injecting thirty pounds' worth of heroin a day and took occasional diazepam. His last heroin hit had been at 06.30hrs; nearly fifteen hours ago.

He had already been interviewed and had asked to see me. Again he claimed that he was "rattling doc"; aching with the snuffles and a headache. But he was fully orientated, his pupils, pulse and blood pressure were all normal. He had no goosebumps or tremor. This was not 'cold turkey'

Despite his demands for something to stop the withdrawal symptoms, I could find no objective evidence of opiate withdrawal. He was also fit to be detained.

I just managed to get home before being called out again. It was almost midnight when I got back to Torquay police station. I was faced with another female. After explaining my role, confidentiality and gaining consent to examine her, she told me that she injected ten pounds' worth heroin a day. She had been on 'benzos', drugs related to diazepam, until six months before and had also been on a methadone programme. She did not touch alcohol and had not had heroin for twenty-four hours. She told me she that she "felt shitty."

Just like the other detainees, she was fully orientated in time and space, her pupils, blood pressure and pulse were all normal and she had no goosebumps, tremor or runny nose. Again I could find no objective evidence of opiate withdrawal. She was either not addicted to heroin or had had a hit more recently than twenty-four hours before.

Ten minutes after I saw her, I was asked to see a man in his thirties, a known schizophrenic. The custody sergeant told me was under specialist care. I still needed to get his consent and explain about confidentiality. He smelt of alcohol and was drowsy; his eyes were half closed. He was on several strong drugs, including injections, every two weeks. His powerful tablets had been given two hours before but he understood why he was there. "I broke a window." The voices had been saying, "I'm going to fucking kill you." He denied taking any street drugs but said he had just drunk two cups of cider.

He let me take his blood pressure. His eyes were not red and, his eye did not flicker when looking to the side; a sign of excess alcohol; known medically as nystagmus.

He was fit to be detained but drowsy which I thought was probably a combination of prescribed medication and alcohol. He would need a psychiatric assessment but that would have to wait until the morning. The drugs and alcohol needed to wear off.

It had not been half an hour since I arrived and I was already on my third case, another young man. He admitted, "I drank too much last night." He claimed the wing mirror of a car had hit him when he was walking down a narrow Devon lane. The allegation was of criminal damage to the wing mirror. Did it hit him or did he hit it? Either way, I was not concerned with the criminal allegation but only with his health.

He also had mental health problems, telling me that he was bipolar. He had been in hospital the previous year and had been taking a drug which prevents the highs and lows of bipolar disorder, for five years but he had stopped taking it three months before.. His regular injections had been stopped a year ago.. Now he was no longer on any medication. Again, he smelt of alcohol and was drowsy. Despite a careful examination, I could not find any injury from the wing mirror. His blood pressure, pulse and eyes were all normal with no nystagmus. He needed to be kept in the cells for the alcohol to wear off, before he could have a psychiatric assessment. I concluded that, this time, it might be that the problem was not drugs but lack of drugs.

It was now half past midnight and, I had spent nearly an hour with the bipolar patient.

Now there was another female to see, this time a possible victim of an assault. When a group of people "kick off" in the street it is impossible for the police to separate victims from assailants; they tend to bring them all in, to preserve the peace.

She was wearing a paper suit when she arrived in the medical room with a female detention officer. After the usual preliminaries, she told me that she was normally well and was not prescribed any medication. She had only drunk three beers. I asked about her last period asI needed to make sure she was not pregnant. She told me that she was menstruating heavily today.

She had been in a scuffle during which she had been hit with a "mallet" on her forehead; was then kicked in the abdomen and the right shoulder, before someone hit her on the right ear. She did not think that she had been knocked out - but could not be certain.

On examination, she had a 2 cms haematoma, a large collection of blood, on her right nostril, with a vertical laceration 0.5 cms long. When I looked in her right ear I could see some blood. The left ear was clear. The right side of her face was tender to the touch but there were no visible injuries.

Even though there was a female detention officer present, understandably, she did not want me to examine the rest of her body.

I made detailed notes, including why I did not document any injuries to her body. Her story fitted the injuries and my evidence might be needed in Court; although anything seen in custody might end up in Court.

I noted that she was fit to be detained. It is not my job to take sides, just note the evidence.

But I still could not go home. At a quarter past three in the morning I saw my sixth patient of the evening. He admitted that had been fighting and his right middle finger was bleeding. I noted a 1 cm long laceration over the dorsum of his PIP joint; the back of the first finger joint. It was a typical fist injury. He told me he was up to date for his tetanus immunization and I dressed the wound with steristrips.

Fifteen minutes later, I saw a police sergeant who had been kneed in the ribs and was now short of breath. He also had pain in his left middle finger. He looked well but he was very tender on the right side of his chest wall in the mid-auxiliary line; directly under his armpit. He had severe pain on springing his ribs, pushing the chest wall in. Listening to his chest it was clear, breath sounds were normal and he moved his rib cage well. His left middle finger was painful with limited flexion.

I explained that he may have fractured ribs but, clinically, there were no internal injuries. I was tired and on "automatic pilot." The Officer was another patient, another person where I had to be objective and not show bias. Working closely with the police there was always a risk that I could feel anger. Why would someone attack an officer who was trying to help? Wasn't he protecting us all from the "bad guys?" But I knew that, even with the police, I was only hearing one side of the story.

At a quarter to four a violent male was brought into the station and taken straight to the cells. It was not safe to go in and so I shouted through the hatch of the cell door, explaining who I was and asking whether he would agree to see me. Sometimes people are willing to see a doctor, even if they hate the police. He was sitting on the cell floor with his back to me.

He shouted back saying he was taking medication but would not give me the name or tell me why he was taking it. All he would say was that he needed in now. He did appear to know where he was and the approximate time. Shouting through the hatch, I explained I could not arrange any medication without knowing what it was. He just kept shouting, "I need my meds." Earlier in my career I might have reacted but the situation was not new. I had dealt with similar characters before. But I had to remain professional. I would always act in the best interests of my "patient", even if the "patient" did not always agree.

For the moment he appeared fit to be detained but I decided that he needed to be on fifteen-minute observations by the police. The question arose whether he was simply an angry drug addict wanting a fix, or whether he was suffering from delirium; part of a serious illness? It was like driving through heavy, fast-moving traffic. I knew the risks; an error of judgement could be serious but I had to concentrate; avoid emotion. Road rage would not help.

I had just arrived home yet again, when the 'phone rang. I arrived back at the nick at five twenty five A young man had been brought in and put straight in the cell. The sergeant was worried. He was "high" on something. He was very alert and over-active but refused to see me. He did tell me that he was not prescribed any medication but admitted he took amphetamines regularly. I could see that his pupils were large but I had no consent for an examination. I could make notes of my observations and decided that he appeared fit to be detained. He had probably taken amphetamines.

I then managed to get home and grab a few hours' sleep, before starting a routine GP surgery at half past eight in the morning.

CHAPTER 1
WHAT AM I DOING HERE?

So why was an ordinary, jobbing GP out of bed in the middle of the night seeing the mad, the bad and the sad, at the local police station?

When I started my GP training in Plymouth, in 1979, I was told, "by the way you will also cover the police". Police work was seen as just an extension of GP practice. The training consisted of "here are your visits. This one's at the police station. Off you go". But suggesting that GP training prepares a young doctor for the work of a police surgeon is as sound as suggesting that GPs can act as anaesthetists because we prescribe sleeping tablets!

I invested in a copy of the large, hard-back book - – *The New Police Surgeon"* - it collected dust as I waded through the other books essential for the trainee GP. I did flick through it before my first police call but failed to get beyond the chapter on the history of the Metropolitan Police.

Throughout my GP training year I was kept busy visiting the police station to take blood from drunk-drivers or to check whether prisoners were fit to be detained. I was even called out to suspicious deaths and examined rape victims. The big gaps in my knowledge were only exposed when I was called to the Plymouth Crown Court, to give evidence in a rape case. After a series of stuttering replies from the witness box, the barrister finally asked me "So, how long have you been qualified, doctor?" It was clear that I was far from being an expert.

However, when I joined my own practice in Torquay, the retiring GP had been a local police surgeon and so I just took over from him.

Devon and Cornwall had an image of a rural idyll by the sea but, with a population of less than two million over forty-five thousand people ended up in police custody every year. Besides sunshine, sand and sea, the restaurants and the hotels, there was another world bubbling away.

Gradually, the police work became a part of my life. On one occasion, I forgot that I was on call for the police and went to the supermarket. This was before the days of mobile 'phones and the police rang my wife at home. I was busy walking down the aisles, looking for soap powder, when the call came over the PA system:, "Would Dr Moore please go to customer services." I suspect that the woman at the desk expected a typical, smart doctor, perhaps in a white coat with a stethoscope around his neck. Instead I wandered up in jeans and t-shirt.

"There's an important call for you, doctor," she said handing me a pen and some paper.

"You've got a police call at Torquay nick," my wife explained. "You've got to come home first to change, so could you also get half a dozen eggs."

I wrote 6 eggs on the piece of paper, which seemed to surprise the woman at customer services. She probably expected details of a medical emergency. I tried to reassure her. "It's OK, I explained. "I'm wanted by the police." I was not sure how much that helped.

Even the seamier side of the work became routine, although the victims of sexual assault did not feel themselves to be just another routine case. One Saturday afternoon, I was watching Torquay United, our local football team, with my sons and, by this time, I had a bleep-pager, which had a screen to tell me the reason for the call. In the middle of the game a call came through.

"Sorry, I've got to go," I explained, "I've got to do a rape." The crowd around us stared at me and my family were, understandably, embarrassed.

After a few years, police officers started asking me to explain the finer details of injuries or whether the examination of a victim of sexual assault fitted in with the story. The work was becoming increasingly professional and I decided that I should either give it up or get properly trained. With negative equity in my house and my surgery and with children heading towards university I needed the money. I was also enjoying the work and so I enrolled on a modular course at Manchester University, with the intriguing acronym "forensic academic group in the north" or FAGIN.

It was only when I started the FAGIN course that I realised just how little I knew. In the first part of the course, on the first module, we were told about consent, confidentiality and the Offences Against the Person Act of 1861. It had not crossed my mind that I did not have a prisoner's consent for an examination if he had not asked to see me and, if I did take a history and examine someone, how much should I tell the police?

There was also a whole world of other ethical aspects. We heard about cases in the Bosnian war when Serbian doctors had signed detailed notes showing no injuries to prisoners, who then arrived at the Red Cross with numerous old injuries. That was extreme but would I ever bias my notes because "we all know he's guilty".

Moreover, it was not only the horrors of the Bosnian War that helped me realise the importance of not taking all police evidence at face value. However, I had learnt to be sceptical long before the FAGIN course.

In my student days, I was hitchhiking with a friend and we were dropped off on a roundabout just off the M4. Soon a police car arrived. Unknown to us, this was not an ordinary roundabout but the intersection of two motorways, one of which was not yet built. Technically, we were pedestrians on a motorway. The officers took our details and allowed us to walk the few hundred yards on the new road to leave the motorway.

When the summons came the police statement claimed that they "saw two people walking along the hard shoulder attempting to thumb a lift". We were guilty of being pedestrians on a motorway, and pleaded guilty but the police version was spun in a way that would have made a politician proud. It is possible that the magistrate was not convinced. We were only fined £3.

Luckily, my offence has never appeared during police vetting procedures. Over the years, I have worked closely with the police and have often been impressed by their integrity but it is sometimes helpful to remember that things are seldom what they seem.

As a police surgeon I had two roles. The first was as a doctor caring for a patient and the other objectively to record forensic evidence. The minor graze, which could be irrelevant to the GP, might hold vital clues in a police investigation. I was also independent from the police. My evidence might, or might not, help their investigations.

Over the years, the job changed. Both prisoners and defence lawyers used the name police surgeon to imply that we were in the pockets of the police. One prisoner told me, "I don't want a police doctor, I want a real doctor." In court, barristers could imply that our evidence was biased. The word "surgeon" was also no longer appropriate. Today people see surgeons as doctors who carry out operations. Police surgeons do not work for the police and are not surgeons. Otherwise, it was a great name. We are now called 'FMEs' or forensic medical examiners.

Today, nurses carry out most of the work in custody centres equally well. My hope is that this book will give the reader some insight into a world of crime which is not only in the rougher parts of large cities but on your doorstep. All the cases are genuine, although names and details have been changed, to maintain confidentiality.

CHAPTER 2

REAL MURDER MOST FOUL

"Death seems to provide the minds of the Anglo-Saxon race with a greater fund of innocent enjoyment than any other single subject."

Dorothy L. Sayers 1934

I was asleep when the phone rang. "We've got a body here, doc. Can you come and take a look?"

I headed out to a local dairy where the milkmen had arrived to load their floats and found a body lying in the courtyard.

Through the heavy morning rain I could see a man's body lying face down over the edge of the pavement. Scenes of crime officers (SOCOs) had protected the area with two cordons of "Police, do not cross" tape and a uniformed officer protected the outer cordon. The crime scene manager showed me the pathway to the body, the area that had already been cleared of any trace evidence. However, with all that rain it was likely that any other evidence had been washed away.

In the past some very senior officers would visit a high profile crime scene, probably hoping they might be photographed or filmed by news crews. The officer in charge of the investigation could not risk his career by pointing out that the boss was damaging trace evidence. Nowadays, a crime scene manager is appointed and, whatever the rank, the manager could override the orders of the Chief Constable or Home Secretary if they affected the crime scene. There is one exception. If there is any possibility that the victim is still alive, we forget trace evidence. Saving a life is more important than any evidence.

In the dairy it looked as though the man had fallen, possibly when drunk, and struck his head on the edge of the pavement. I looked for any injuries, although examining injuries on dead bodies can be misleading. If someone is killed instantly the external injury can appear small. The heart stops and so the bruising or bleeding does not develop. Again, I have seen in detective fiction, the "expert" looking at a body and commenting "that's too small to have caused death". No it isn't.

Bruising is also controversial. Bruising is caused by bleeding under the skin, but to spread under the skin blood requires circulation and so true bruising will not occur after death, although the skin can be damaged, leaving marks, which are easily mistaken for a bruise.

Post mortem livido, or staining of the body, was over the corpse's front, implying that he had not been moved after death. People who have never seen a dead body, which is most people, will sometimes panic when they first see one. "He's covered in bruises!" they say. However, after death, the heart stops and blood settles where gravity dictates; in the dependent parts. If someone died on his back, then the back, neck, arms and legs will show "post mortem staining"; a purple-pink colour.

The post mortem would tell us more. All I could do was to confirm that he was dead. A junior officer then asked the question every senior detective knows is unanswerable, "how long has he been dead, doc?"

The expert in crime fiction also looks at the body and proclaims that he died at 12.43 hrs. If the person was seen walking around and chatting at 20.00 hrs and was found dead at 08.00 hrs I can say with confidence that he died between those times. Beyond that it gets difficult.

However, he had post mortem staining, which occurs three to six hours after death and is fixed after eight hours.

And there was no *rigor mortis*, stiffening of the body. There is a simple rule of thumb that suggests that *rigor* starts after six hours, takes another six hours to be fully established and disappears after another twelve hours. But this has massive variations. An even simpler rule, which even I could remember in the middle of the night, was that if a body is warm and flaccid it has probably been dead for less than half a day, if it is cold and flaccid it is probably more than two days. This does not produce an exact time as sometimes given in detective fiction but it does produce a more accurate result.

The post mortem confirmed that death had resulted from a head injury but it was not until the police made further enquires that the true situation became clear.

As the body was found in a dairy the investigation was called Operation Friesian. Once the man was identified, the police visited his flat and a neighbour told them that two men lived in the flat. Overnight, they heard shouting and the noise of a possible fight. By the time the police tried to trace the other men, they had fled to Thailand.

I was one of several witnesses to give evidence at the formal extradition hearing. The men were then arrested by the Thai police but formal extradition was not needed. After a short time in a Thai jail they agreed to return voluntarily.

It turned out that the two men were drug dealers and the deceased owed them money. They beat him up in the flat, put him in the back of their van and dumped the body at the dairy. They were both convicted of murder and sentenced to life imprisonment.

In the same week, I was called to a body outside the theatre on Torquay seafront. Again the weather was poor and it initially looked like an accident. Had a drunk fallen over? However, the area was sealed and treated as a crime scene.

After a few days, a young man arrived at the police station. He had been out drinking with some friends on the night of the murder and had witnessed one of the group, known to be violent, attack the victim because he was gay. The witness was terrified in case he would put himself in danger by coming forward. However, he could not live with the guilt. After the arrest, others came forward. Eventually the murderer was given a life sentence; to the relief of all the witnesses.

I had seen the scenes of two murders in a week and had, initially, put both down to natural causes. Watching a television detective story (just after these two cases), in which there was a horrific murder, my teenage son commented: "Don't worry. Dad would say it was natural causes."

The public image of murder from detective novels and television "who-dun-its" is far from the real thing. In most real murders there is no debate over "who dun it". We know who killed the victim. It is rarely Miss Scarlet in the library with the lead pipe. It was not my role to become an amateur sleuth. All I ever needed to do was to confirm death, although officers often bounced ideas off me.

The law surrounding the definition of death is vague. Only a doctor can certify death. Put simply, "you're not dead until I say so". A coroner once pointed out to me that this also means you are dead when the doctor says so. What would happen if a doctor wrongly certifies someone and the relatives register the death? For example, conditions such as hypothermia and some overdoses can give rise to the appearance of death. There is no legal system in place to reverse a registration of death, so what would happen, could "the deceased" pick up their life insurance personally?

In the 1980s and 1990s the duty police surgeon was called out to every unexplained death. This included suicides. There were several occasions when I was called to a railway line to see the remains of someone who had jumped in front of a train but the police statement could only say he "appeared to be dead." I was even called to Brixham harbour to certify a headless body which had come up with fishing nets out at sea. According to the police she "appeared to be dead."

Most of the dead bodies I saw were eventually found to have resulted from natural causes. Fortunately, murder and even suicide are not the commonest causes of death.

One elderly lady went for a walk on her own and disappeared. Finally, her body was found in a wood behind a local petrol station. When I arrived there was no sign of the police or of a body; just a queue waiting to pay for their petrol. I went into the shop but, rather than join the queue I asked the cashier, "I'm a doctor. I understand the police are here and need me?" It was the most tactful phraseology I could manage.

"Oh, if you've come to see the dead body it's round the back," she shouted over the queue. The elderly lady was dead and it turned out to be the result of natural causes.

One hot, summer day I was called out of surgery to visit a typical, Victorian, terraced house. The elderly man who lived there alone had not been seen for several weeks. The police had broken in, to find the floor sticky and the man's body on a chair, decomposing in the kitchen. I managed to certify death without going too close and felt grateful that I was not the undertaker.

There was another case where the body was not easy to examine I was called in the night. There had been a fire. The fire brigade had successfully put the fire out but, in the lounge, there was a hole in the floor. Underneath the lounge was a storeroom, which opened into the garden. At the back of the storeroom, under the hole in the lounge floor was a body. Again, all I needed to do was to certify him. After a full investigation it turned out that he had fallen asleep with his pipe still lit. He had also had a heart attack, which probably killed him before the fire.

In a field outside Brixham, a member of the public noticed a portion of backbone sticking out of a bank. It was, again, at night. When I arrived the police had erected lights and I could just see that half way down a typical Devon bank on the edge of the field a portion of spinal column was protruding. There were also pieces of a black plastic sack in which the "body" appeared to have been buried. The spine was small and did not look human.

"Could it be a baby?" asked the officer.

"Highly unlikely."

"But can you be absolutely, one hundred per cent certain?

Nothing in medicine is that certain. We started to dig, aware that, in the unlikely event that this was a baby, we would need trace evidence. There were also plenty of maggots and so the burial was fairly recent. There is a whole speciality of forensic entomology, concerned with assessing how long a body has been left, by examining the maggots – not a specialism that would appeal to everyone. After about fifteen minutes, a decomposing dog's head could be seen.

It is likely that someone buried their pet dog in the field where he used to enjoy his walks. Unfortunately it was not buried deep enough.

Any bodily decomposition requires oxygen. In some soils a coffin can keep oxygen out, slowing or even stopping decomposition. In Bram Stoker's *Dracula* a coffin is opened to reveal the body of a girl with no sign of decomposition but, as soon as the sun strikes the body, she starts to decompose. This was supposed to be clear evidence that she was a vampire but, more mundanely, it is just evidence that the coffin was airtight.

It was rare to find only parts of bodies and even rarer for the police to ask for my opinion on them. Luckily, I was not available when they found a hand on the banks of the River Dart. A local GP looked at it and declared that it was genuine. The hand was sealed in an evidence bag and taken to the pathologist. The police then started a massive search for the rest of the body and even sent the helicopter up. It was only when the hand reached the pathologist that they realised the hand was plastic. It had been bought at the local joke shop.

Today when a body is found sanity has prevailed. If it is clear that the victim is dead, the police simply call the scenes of crime officers (SOCOs), assuming the victim is human. If there is any sign of life, the paramedics are called; if not they secure the scene. With trace evidence becoming increasingly sensitive, the forensic investigators do not want the FMEs walking around and damaging vital clues. In one case, in the 1980s, an FME trod on a flowerbed but did not tell the officers. Several weeks were wasted as the murder enquiry tried to find a match for the footprint.

So, why did I miss two murders in a week? The body and even the post mortem are only a part of an investigation. The police need to look at three pieces of evidence: the person's history, the crime scene and the post mortem. With these three the story can usually be pieced together. In both of my cases it was the history that provided the key. FMEs need to be slightly obsessional when taking the history. This is as important as the crime scene or post mortem.

The body of a man was found in his newly refurbished flat in Manchester. He had suffered from chronic obstructive pulmonary disease, a serious lung condition and was well known to his GP and the local hospital. Normally the GP would have written a death certificate but he was on holiday. Legally, in England, a doctor can only write a death certificate if he or she has seen the patient alive within the last two weeks. The case had to be referred to the coroner who ordered a post mortem. This confirmed his lung problems as well as serious heart disease.

The pathologist was prepared to accept that death had resulted from "natural causes" – until his assistant made an off-the-cuff comment. "It's a pity about his dog." Apparently, as well as his body, there was also the body of a dog found in the flat. The dog had already been cremated but the pathologist checked the elderly man for carbon monoxide poisoning; was there a problem with the gas supply to the newly refurbished flats? The levels were high. The flats were checked and found to have high carbon monoxide levels. All the residents were at risk. They were all moved to temporary accommodation and, before being sued, the building company went out of business.

There would have been more deaths if the GP had not been on holiday, if the patient had not had a dog and if the pathologist's assistant had not been told, by chance, that the dog had also died.

The scene is also crucial. First, one takes an overview: where is the body in the room, what is the position, is there any evidence of an apparent fall, is there anything remarkable about the clothing or the furniture? Today this is all noted by the SOCOs and photographed but, when I was working, in the 1980s and 90s, it was vital that I made such notes. If I fell short of a good standard, I could easily end up, facing a barrister in the Crown Court in several months or even a year's time, explaining (for example), why my evidence was at odds with evidence from the police.

The overview can be misleading. When an elderly person starts to die from the cold -, hypothermia -, they actually feel hot. In some cases, they even start to undress. Finding an elderly lady, dead, with her skirt and knickers around her ankles, can look as though a sexual assault might have taken place. Again, we need information from a post mortem and the history as well as more details from the scene to decide the cause of death.

The onset of sudden death from a pulmonary embolus, which is a blood clot on the lung, can be accompanied by a sudden desire to defecate. Accordingly, someone who has had a sudden massive pulmonary embolus might have pulled his trousers down.

I once saw a dead, elderly man who lived alone, with his trousers down, kneeling, facing the toilet. By his side was a "top shelf girlie" magazine open at a picture of a naked model. The post mortem found that he had suffered a massive heart attack. As death clearly resulted from natural causes, why cause more grief to the family by speculating?

There may be obvious clues, such as a syringe and other drug-taking paraphernalia or some evidence of suicide. However, some clues are less obvious and are easily missed. Before, we used to look for a build-up of milk bottles on the doorstep, as a clue to time of death but not many people have milk delivered any more. However, the date on a newspaper or franking marks on post on the mat might help in a similar way.

So why is the scene so important? We need to go back to Edmund Locard (1877-1966), a doctor and lawyer working in Lyon He was a real life 'Sherlock Holmes' of France and the founder of modern, forensic science. His principle is summed up as "every contact leaves a trace." If I touch a knife some material from my hand will be on the knife and some material from the knife will be on my hand.

When still a medical student, Locard developed an interest in the application of science to investigating crime; today we call it forensic science.

In 1910 the Lyon police department helped him set up the first "police laboratory" in the world. This was only a few attic rooms, but he managed to collect evidence from crime scenes and examine them scientifically. Finally, in 1912, his laboratory was officially recognised by the police.

During the Great War he continued his forensic work, this time working for the French secret service, trying to find out the location and cause of death of soldiers and prisoners, from the clues in the stains and damage to their uniforms.

Today trace evidence lies at the heart of forensic science. After a serious crime, the SOCOs examine the scene slowly and systematically. This takes time. In a double murder investigation in Torquay the SOCOs took several days, locking the house up at night and returning the next day.

The first job is to create a clear pathway to the body. One area is examined first and anyone approaching the body must use this path. Unlike in television dramas, we do not walk around the body scratching our chins.

Even on carpet shoes can leave a foot print. There may be hair fibres or saliva. Some burglars have been known to take a bite out of a piece of cheese leaving both their dental impression and their DNA. In the Soham murders of two young school girls, the bodies were dumped on an overgrown path in the countryside. A botanist managed to calculate how long it had taken the weeds to grow back and, therefore, how long ago the bodies had been dumped.

In another case, the body of a baby was found buried in some peat. The peat was analysed and found to be unique to Estonia. Enquires at all the local garden centres found that only one sold peat from Estonia. A search of their records uncovered a suspect who had bought the peat and the case ended in a conviction.

My brother, a detective inspector, had another case, in which a few tiny fragments of glass were found at a murder scene. A rent collector had been attacked and killed. When examined, the glass was found to be from a pair of spectacles. The prescription turned out to be unusual. The owner of the spectacles in question had astigmatism. Asking around the local opticians, the lens was matched with a customer who had left the area immediately after the murder. He was traced, found and arrested. Apparently, he had taken off his spectacles and put them in his top pocket, before attacking the victim. The victim had hit back, smashing the glasses. The murderer thought he had picked up all the pieces.

There is a belief that all will be answered in the post mortem but, as several cases above have shown, the post mortem can be unhelpful or even misleading. It is only one piece of the jigsaw puzzle.

Despite its limitations, in England and Wales, every coroner's case requires a post mortem. As a result, we probably do too many, too quickly. Having a smaller number of post mortems carried out only when there are real concerns about the cause of death might result in a more productive approach.

The mass murderer, Dr Shipman, literally got away with murder, when pathologists did not send away samples for toxicology. But they had no reason to do so, because no one suspected the GP of killing his patients with doses of diamorphine.

Even if samples are taken for analysis, drug levels found in the system after death may be misleading. Steven Karch a forensic pathologist from California argues that "dead people are different". How accurately do post mortem blood samples reflect the levels of substances present in the blood in life? The experts rely on research into how drugs are broken down in the body but this research is carried out on the living, not the dead. We cannot, actually, assume that the apparent level of a drug in a dead body reflects the level in life. For a start, when the circulation stops, any drug present will simply defuse through the tissues. Bacteria can also affect drug levels and can even *increase* the amount of pure morphine. We often hear argument in Coroner's and Crown Courts that the level of a drug in a body was 'therapeutic' or 'lethal'. While the technology for measuring sub-nanograms of drugs has improved enormously, our understanding of the results has not.

Today many FMEs are full-time but, in the 1980s and 90s, because I was a GP by day and police surgeon by night, occasionally, I saw my patients in the police station. In one embarrassing moment, I shook a very drunk man, who was lying on the cell floor and asked him "who's your normal doctor?"

"You are." came the reply. He was more conscious than I had realised.

Although working as the accused's own GP can be useful it can also lead to a conflict of interest.

A twenty five year old man, called Aaron, joined my list in the late 1990s, having moved down from Manchester. He told me that he was a heroin addict but was trying to withdraw. I may have been slightly sceptical because no heroin addict will admit that they want to continue. But there were some positive signs. He had held down a job overseas for six months before heroin took over his life and he already had an appointment with the drugs' team. However positive it all seemed, I was not going to prescribe until I had checked his story with his last GP and whether he really had the appointment with the drugs' team.

It turned out that he was genuine. I prescribed methadone for daily, supervised consumption at the local pharmacist, on the advice of the drugs' team. A week later I saw him and prescribed methadone again, once more under supervised consumption.

The following day two police officers came to see me. Aaron's flat mate was in the local intensive care unit with severe injuries to his neck inflicted with a kitchen knife. He had been out with Aaron in the evening, drunk a large amount of alcohol and smoked cannabis. On returning to the flat a fight broke out.

Aaron was now on the run and the police wanted to know whether he was taking medication. Would he need to see a doctor for a new prescription? I took legal advice. Could I tell the police or was his medical history confidential? I was advised that my duty to protect the public outweighed my duty of confidentially. I told the officers that he had been prescribed two weeks' of medication but he could only get it from the local chemist in person. The last dose would be wearing off and, unless Aaron could persuade another doctor to prescribe, he would soon be suffering from withdrawal symptoms.

The next day I was asked to see him at Torquay police station. He had been arrested in Plymouth, thirty miles away. He had not had any methadone for fifty hours and he was clearly withdrawing. I prescribed a substitute and arranged to see him again. He was not well enough to agree to give samples or to be interviewed. If we had gone ahead a defence lawyer could then have argued that he had not given informed consent, making the consequential evidence inadmissible.

Two hours later he had improved. I examined him in the presence of a police officer and scenes of crime officer. I also made sure he gave written consent. He had to understand that I was not longer acting as his GP although I was still independent and not acting for the police.

There were some grazes over his hands and lower back. I took scrapings from underneath his nails and also sent some nail cuttings away. If he had scratched the victim there might be evidence under the nails. I also took a blood sample for DNA profiling and drugs' testing. In the late 1990s, we used blood, rather than mouth swabs, for DNA.

Later on in the same evening, I was at the custody centre, when the news came through that the victim had died. It was now a murder enquiry.

In November, nine months after the death, I gave evidence at Exeter Crown Court. The defence barrister asked me whether Aaron was a good patient; did he really want to come off drugs, did he turn up for his appointment? The answer was yes. The question for the court was did he mean to kill or was it a tragic accident?

Under English common law, the elements of murder are: "the unlawful killing by someone of sound mind, of a human being, under the Queen's peace, with malice aforethought, either express or implied." In Henry 1st's day the victim had to be a Frenchman or foreigner.

Surprisingly it does not require malice or aforethought. It would be no defence to argue that Aaron and his flat mate were friends and so there could not be any malice and aforethought does not mean that a murder must be pre-planned days in advance. Aforethought means that there must be an intention to kill or cause grievous (i.e. really serious) bodily harm at the time of the incident. This begs the question "what is meant by intention?" If I push the wrong person off a cliff could I argue that I did not intend to kill that particular person? No one can get away with murder that easily. Intention means that death or serious injury is a virtually certain consequence. If the "wrong" person is killed, it is still murder because there has been a transfer of malice.

Likewise, if a terrorist plants a bomb in a shopping centre, timed to go off on a Saturday afternoon, it is "virtually certain" that people will be killed. It is murder even though the terrorist did not know who was going to be killed. The drug dealers who committed the murder at the start of this chapter may not have set out to kill their victim but their assault was so vicious that death was "virtually certain."

Until 1996 the death had to occur within a year and a day from the commission of the act but, because of the benefits of modern, critical care, this was changed. Now there must just be a direct link between the act and the death.

The jury did not believe that Aaron had "malice aforethought" and, eventually, he was acquitted of murder but found guilty of manslaughter. He was sentenced to five years in prison.

In most cases we can establish the identity of the body. But, occasionally, this can be a problem. There are obvious methods such as identity cards and passports; appearance; race; hair colour; tattoos; scars, and gender but let's suppose that we are still unsure.

X-rays might reveal past injuries or operations, perhaps an artificial hip or a metal work around an old fracture. A forensic odontologist can assess the teeth and, hopefully, match them to dental records.

However, DNA is now the most well known. It might be matched with samples from a possible victim. In one case a charred body from an aircraft disaster had the DNA matched with some material from the victim's comb which was found in her home. Or it may be matched with samples from family members. DNA from the bones of the last Tsar of Russia and the Romanov family, was matched with that from living relatives, including the Duke of Edinburgh. Of course, it was the DNA of matrilineal descendants which showed how a skeleton, found in a Leicester car park, belonged to King Richard III.

Sometimes, despite all the investigations, we fail to identify a body. One evening, a well-dressed, Asian man booked into a large Torquay hotel. He looked like a successful businessman. He paid in cash in advance and was generous with his tips.

The following morning he did not appear. When the hotel maid entered his room he was dead. There was no sign of any trauma, the room was tidy. Despite a thorough search of all his possessions, there was no evidence of his identity.

Post mortem and toxicology found that he had died of cyanide poisoning, a very unusual cause of death. His DNA did not appear on any data base. Racially he was believed to be from southern India or Sri Lanka. He was circumcised, which implied that he might be a Muslim. A large, international investigation found nothing; which was probably his aim. Some terrorists carry cyanide capsules in case they are caught but he had not been caught. Another possibility was that he had been involved in the Tamil Tigers, fallen out with the leaders and then killed himself? There was no evidence that anyone else was involved in his death.

He was buried with no name. We will probably never know who he was or exactly what happened to him and that is probably what he wanted.

Murder and sudden death is less exciting in real life than in fiction. Agatha Christie, who also came from Torquay, was a great writer of fiction but I have never seen a Hercule Poirot or Miss Marple in real life. Police officers are far more intelligent than Agatha Christie's Inspector Japp or Sherlock Holmes's Inspector Lestrade. In court many murder cases hinge on whether the killing was intended or accidental. There was a fight, someone was killed but was the killing a tragic accident; and so manslaughter – or even in lawful self-defence?

CHAPTER 3
I CANNOT FACE TOMORROW

"The instant he saw the word "funeral "he felt this was where everything that had gone before had led him, and he decided that he couldn't face tomorrow".

Alastair Campbell's novel "All in the mind" p275

Not every sudden death is murder. Sometimes I was called to sudden deaths from natural causes but most were suicides. Unlike the FMEs today, in the 1980s and 1990s I was called to every suspicious death.

It was rare to see hardened policemen close to tears; they usually managed scepticism in the most difficult situations. Therefore, when on one occasion, I arrived to find an officer's attempt at the stiff upper lip beginning to crumble I was not sure what I was going to find. It was the middle of a hot summer's night at a beauty spot overlooking the Bay.

In the car park was a new car, parked to overlook the sea. The windows and doors were now open. It was a still night. The smell of exhaust fumes still hung in the air.

The senior officer took me over to the car and shone a torch into the front seats. A young couple, probably in their 20s, were lying with their arms around each other. They had been dead for a few hours and were cold, with pink skin caused by carbon monoxide poisoning. On the back seat were presents wrapped carefully and labelled, along with a note.

My job was to confirm what everyone already knew; that they were dead. There did not appear to be any suspicious circumstances.

Later investigations found that they were a young couple who had run up serious debts. Unable to face either family and ashamed of the situation, they hired a car, drove down to Devon and killed themselves, while playing music, overlooking the sea. Not only had they left a note for their families but they had bought presents, which were carefully wrapped.

I felt a strange mixture of tragedy and anger. Money is only man made; there must have been a better way out of their problems.

Young lovers' killing themselves, following social pressure, probably pre-dates Romeo and Juliet.

Suicide following the ending of romantic relationships seems to strike a chord with the public. In a review of three hundred and six operas, there were seventy seven suicides, seven of which included a murder, followed by suicide. Puccini wrote twelve operas, between 1884 and 1924, of which four contained a suicide. This reflects real life. A study, in 1965, found that a third of all murders were followed by the suicide of the perpetrator; the same proportion as in fictional opera over the centuries.

Until 1961 the young lovers' car would have been a crime scene; suicide was then a crime and we still talk about "committing" suicide.

I never spoke to the families of this tragic couple but I suspect that they would have had no idea of their plans. Suicide can, sometimes, be predicted but some people keep their emotions hidden, especially men.

I was once called to a lake in a nearby park. The police had found a body. It was that of a local businessman, who had told his family that he had a meeting in London. He had even bought the train tickets. His wife assumed that he was still in London when his body was dragged from the lake. It turned out that he had left home, taken an overdose and then jumped in the lake.

In both these cases I did not know the victims but could still feel the tragedy and their deaths seemed pointless.

Suicides triggered by romance are usually one-sided. I felt the same emotions of tragedy and anger in a case which touched on my work as a GP and as a FME but, as the suicide's GP, I also felt personal guilt. Could I have done more?

Dean Reeves was a patient of mine. He appeared happily married and was devoted to his three children. However, his wife, Janice, had slowly fallen out of love. She did not hate her husband but, emotionally, there was nothing there. Should she stay and live the lie or move on? Not long after she told Dean that the marriage was over, he was found in his car in a lay-by with a hosepipe attached to the exhaust. He was rescued and admitted to hospital.

Janice came to see me. She still cared for Dean, although she was no longer in love with him. However she also knew that, if she left, he would try to kill himself again. This time he might be successful. She made the decision that she would not be blackmailed. She had to live her own life.

A few weeks later, I was called out by the police. As I arrived, I recognised Dean's van. His boss had gone home and Dean had promised to lock up. Instead, he had taken the van to a closed yard, blocked all the vents and attached a hosepipe to the exhaust. He was dead in the driving seat. I recognised the photos of Janice and the children on his lap. I knew and Janice knew that, if he had managed to survive the emotional trauma of the break, his life would have moved on but he did not survive.

I was left with the feeling that I should have been able to prevent this tragedy. Somehow, suicide appears different from other deaths. If every possible treatment is offered to a patient with terminal cancer or severe heart disease, their death is sad but, somehow, inevitable. Everything possible has been done. But, as his GP, could I have prevented Dean's death? I knew he was at high risk but he had made up his mind. Was there anything we could have done short of locking him up forever?

Were both Dean and the young couple mentally ill or had they made a rational decision? There is a difference between true clinical depression and unhappiness. It is normal to be unhappy after a break up, bereavement or when heavily in debt. In contrast clinical depression is not founded on logical problems; it is just a condition in which everything looks bleak. However, one third of suicides are carried out by people who are not clinically depressed, just unhappy.

Although the risk of suicide is difficult to assess there were some situations which rang alarm bells.

A middle aged man was brought in by a patrol car. He had been driving erratically through the narrow Devon lanes and was pulled over because the officers thought that he may have been drinking. He was sober but, in the car he had a bottle of whisky and a packet of sleeping pills. In the boot was a hosepipe.

When I saw him he was withdrawn; he just wanted to die. The only reason he was still alive was that he could not find a hidden field to pull over and gas himself. There had been 'travellers' in the area and so the farmers had locked their gates and placed boulders across the entrances. In this case the psychiatrist agreed to immediate admission under the Mental Health Act. If there had been no 'travellers' threatening to set up in the farmer's fields he would have been dead.

And so an important question to ask someone who may be suicidal is "what's stopping you?" Sometimes, the patient smiles and says: "I wouldn't do that to my family." In one case, a depressed patient said that he would never kill himself because of his dog. He then told me that the dog was aged fifteen. I wondered whether we should get him a puppy.

Luckily I never faced the nightmare of a suicide in the cells. But this was just luck. A common call out to the police station was to see whether someone was at risk of suicide; either having been brought in following a crime or under the Mental Health Act. This often meant making a joint assessment, working with a social worker and psychiatrist.

As a GP I could not always prevent a suicide even though I knew the patient, the family and the social background. I also had the notes. I had none of these advantages, with a stranger, in the police station, out of hours.

The first question to ask was "is the patient mentally ill?" Suicide is no longer a crime and, in a free society, sane people are entitled make up their own minds, within the law.

Here I heard both sides of the argument. In one case the psychiatrist arranged for a man to be admitted under the Mental Health Act even though he had made a rational decision to kill himself. Trying to take your own life, he argued, was such a serious and irrational act that he must have a mental illness.

In another case, a different psychiatrist argued that such a patient was clear and rational. Suicide was not against the law and so he should be released. The custody sergeant was not happy. If he was released from police custody and immediately killed himself legally it would become a death "after contact with the Police". These are usually investigated by the Independent Police Complaints Commission (IPPC). There would also have to be a coroner's inquest and, inevitably, the question would be asked "why did the police let him go?" The media find it easier to blame the police, rather than the psychiatrist. One would have to argue that it was the patient's choice and that the police and mental health services could not stop him. If kept in custody, against his will, the police would be in breach of the European Convention on Human Rights, Article 5; the right to liberty. However, if he were released to kill himself, might they be in breach of Article 2, securing the right to life?

I once asked a psychiatrist whether we could have a questionnaire for patients to enable us to assess suicide risk. Sadly it is so unpredictable that any questionnaire might be dangerous; giving the professionals a false sense of security. Suicidal feelings are the result of a complicated mixture of social, physical and psychological factors. The National Institute for Health and Clinical Excellence (NICE) has recommended that none of the simple risk-assessment tools should be used on their own. They are all unreliable.

So I was left with a problem. How was I to assess the risk, if called out in the night to see someone who might be at risk of suicide? There were some factors making suicide more likely: recent divorce, separation or debt as with these tragic cases mentioned above. I also knew that the risk increases with age and is three times more common in men than women, although women are more likely to make a gesture without meaning to kill themselves; para-suicide. .

Without the patient's notes or access to the GP, I had no idea whether they were being treated for depression or even whether they had just walked out of hospital; I had to rely on the patient. Clinical depression is an illness which is not the same as simple unhappiness. It does respond to treatment, although this can take several weeks to be effective. There was no quick fix at the police station. Depression is always difficult to diagnose in a stranger.

I could ask whether they, or any of their family, had attempted suicide in the past. Previous suicide attempts increase the risk of future suicide.

Since pending legal proceedings can also create a suicide risk, anyone arrested and locked in a cell could be at risk, which is why every prisoner is searched and shoe laces and belts are removed.

In general practice we tried to create a medical summary for our patients, coding each condition into the computer. One of the codes was "successful suicide attempt", which left me wondering why the patient was still on our list.

I also realised that drug addicts are more likely than others to commit suicide as well as more likely to kill themselves with an accidental overdose.

Even successful treatment of depression carries a suicide risk. When severely depressed, patients lose motivation; just sit and look at the wall but, as they improve, motivation returns before mood improves. They still want to die and, as the treatment starts to work, they gain the motivation to take action. The highest risk of suicide is as depressive people improve with treatment and some treatments can even increase the risk of suicide in the long term. One group of anti-depressants increases suicide risk in people under the age of 18.

Accordingly, the police have to be vigilant with every detainee. Everyone is thoroughly searched. Some prisoners are monitored through CCTV in the cell; some are even put in paper suits and very high risk ones on "cell watch", with an officer sitting, watching all the time.

Prisoners could be let out into the yard, an outside area surrounded by bars to allow for exercise and fresh air, but they are monitored with CCTV. In one police station I recall that the sergeant looked at the yard CCTV to see a pair of feet dangling. He pressed the emergency button and raced to the yard to find the prisoner doing pull- up on the roof bars. He was more interested in keeping fit than hanging himself!

Another risk factor is a past history of sexual abuse. The problem here is that people may not admit to being a victim. They often feel guilty, as though it is somehow their fault. They may believe that they have moved on and are afraid to open up the emotional wounds.

When I saw a very disturbed young woman lying in a cell, with numerous scars from attempted self harm, I was almost certain that she was the victim of sexual abuse. She had learning difficulties and serious mental health problems. She had tried to assault someone but we had a more serious problem. She had wrapped up razor blades and pushed them inside her vagina. We could not leave her in the cell. She could self-harm at any time. Any attempt to retrieve them, even if ethical and legal, would have been dangerous.

She was also hearing voices, or rather one voice. Her "voice" was called Cheryl. I joined the detention officer who was sitting with her in the cell. For over an hour we spoke to her. It was "Cheryl" who had told her where to put the razor blades. We gentle pointed out that Cheryl now wanted them out. Cheryl was not happy any longer and wanted her to give the blades to me. Gradually, one by one, the blades were removed. Physical wounds heal but emotional scars are for life.

Some victims of abuse lead successful lives but the emotional scars are always under the surface. This can lead to suicide, even after many years.

Julie Lang was one of my GP patients. She was a successful social worker in her mid thirties. Her notes were thin. I only knew her for the occasional appointment for family planning and a visit to the surgery with the children. This time she had been persuaded to come to the surgery; a visit she seemed to see as either pointless or dangerous, I was not sure which.

"My line manager told me that I had to come for help. I may be wasting your time."

She had been discussing a case of child sex abuse with a senior social worker when she mentioned that she understood; not because of any course or training but because she had been there. A "friend" of the family had sexually abused her throughout her childhood. He had insisted that this was "our little secret" and she had not told anyone. She also felt "guilty" and "dirty", blaming herself.

She was successful at school, went to University and, eventually, qualified as a social worker. The "little secret" in her childhood had been kept secret. The hurt and pain was still there but she had managed to lock it in an imaginary box and get on with life.

When she mentioned the abuse, her line manager followed the received wisdom. This is not something you should keep bottled up. If you open the box, the evil will be exorcised. If not, it will always be there; nagging in the background, creating difficulties in everyday life. Clearly, she needed specialist counselling.

When I saw her she discussed the fact of the abuse without any details. It was as though she were discussing a remote client. I colluded in her unemotional, factual account and said I would arrange specialist counselling.

I did not see her for several weeks although the counsellor sent me a formal letter simply stating that she was taking her onto her case-load.

When I did see Julie next, she had lost her sparkle; her eyes seemed dim and she avoided eye contact. She still did not want to discuss any details but simply wanted "something to help me sleep".

Any attempt to ask open questions and talk in more detail was met with monosyllable answers. Maybe she was right; she was already receiving counselling and did not need any intrusion from me. However, I could see that she had slipped into a true, depressive illness. I started her on a course of anti-depressants, hoping that they would be more effective than potentially addictive sleeping pills. I also suggested that she take some time off work. She had a stressful job and could not deal with the emotional traumas of her clients in the state she was in herself.

"It will only be for a week or two; just to catch your breath" I suggested naively.

After the consultation I was worried, but my GP partners said they would have managed the case in exactly the same way. Perhaps her depression was the pain coming out. It was like bursting an abscess. It may be painful when the knife goes in but the pus needs to come out before any cure.

I saw Julie regularly over the next few weeks. The "pus" may have been draining but she was not improving. I then noticed that, despite the hot summer day, she was wearing long sleeves and kept pulling them down. When I mentioned it she said it was nothing, but there were superficial cuts on her left wrist. There was only one explanation. She had started to harm herself.

"Do you mind if I talk to your counsellor?" I asked. "Just to make sure we're all pulling in the same direction." She agreed. I am not sure whether she realised that I had spotted her cuts. If she did she did not acknowledge anything. The stakes had just risen and she needed specialist help.

The counsellor agreed that she was deteriorating. She had also noticed the cuts and said that she would discuss the case with the consultant psychiatrist.

The letter from the psychiatrist suggested a specialist anti-depressant at a high dose. He also arranged to see her regularly. I received regular letters from the mental health team but the self-harm was getting worse. She was not making any progress.

I then received a phone call from the psychiatrist. "I've just seen Julie in the clinic," he explained. "She's much worse, marked suicidal ideation. I'm going to have to admit her. She agreed so we don't have to section her under the Mental Health Act." That was a small relief. How would it affect her career as a senior social worker if she had been sectioned under the Mental Health Act? Moreover, she was going to get the care she needed.

The next day I got another call; she had changed her mind and was trying to walk out. The nursing staff had placed her on a section 5 (a), meaning that she could not leave but had to be assessed by two doctors within 6 hours.

When I arrived at the hospital she was dressed and looking "distant." She answered in monosyllables and was evasive when I asked specifically about her desire to kill herself. She was clearly at risk and I agreed to sign the form, so that she would have to stay in hospital under a section 3. Technically, this lasts up to six months but is usually discharged much earlier. She seemed to understand.

It was during my evening surgery that I received a phone call from the psychiatrist. After I had seen her, she was taken to her room and left by the staff. Half an hour later, a nurse went in to check on her. She had hanged herself. Her desire to commit suicide had been successful despite the Mental Health Act section.

At the inquest the psychiatrist explained that all patients had to be treated with dignity and respect. As a part of rehabilitation they were given some freedom. To be on continual watch would make any depression worse. It is a difficult balance which, in this case, had gone tragically wrong.

And so, even in hospital, under specialist care, suicides do occur. If we see depression as a potentially fatal illness should we expect one hundred per cent success? No cardiologist expects every patient to survive every heart attack but works to reduce the risk.

My FME work was either prevention of suicide in the cells or picking up the pieces after the event.

When called simply to confirm a death, hanging was common and could be from a low level. These are always traumatic as they are usually found by a member of the family. It is always dangerous in medicine to use the word "always" but, in the cases I saw, hanging was always a suicide. To murder someone by hanging them requires strength and, probably, a whole lynch mob.

Luckily judicial hanging had been stopped by the time I qualified but, when carried out with scientific efficiency, death occurs instantly, as the odontoid process, a bone in the upper neck, pushes through the spinal cord. However, until the 1890s, for many hangings, death was through strangulation.

When working in an Accident and Emergency department I saw a patient who decided to hang himself but left the rope too long. He jumped and broke his ankle.

Overdoses are common but often made it to hospital and so I was not called.

It was not always clear that a body was a suicide. In one case the body was in a flat with knife wounds in the chest. There was chaos and a dagger which would not have looked out of place in an Agatha Christie film. We were concerned that this was a murder scene but it turned out to be suicide; although suicide by self-stabbing through the heart is rare in the UK. At the time I was studying for an exam and needed ten cases for my dissertation. This was ideal. As I left, the officer outside the door turned to me.

"Are you OK, doc?" I grinned. "Yes, I really enjoyed that." This was not the best comment in front of the journalists and the small crowd outside.

If we accept that suicide can be a tragic consequence of clinical depression why do we not treat it in the same way as other illnesses? As well as using the term "committing" suicide, as though it is still a crime, every suicide is considered to be "violent or unnatural" and so has to be reported to the coroner. The coroner has to investigate every case and, in every case, there must be a post mortem examination and an inquest. The facts must be made public. As we now accept that depression in an illness which, like heart disease or cancer, can be fatal why does every case need to be investigated and made public?

Suicide no longer has the stigma of the past but it still seems a pointless tragedy. Why didn't anyone do anything? Surely the young couple who killed themselves could have found a better way out of their problems. Were they both mentally ill or was this a social tragedy? Suicide, like so much in clinical forensic medicine, is complicated and controversial. We no longer believe the suicidal are bad but are they mad or sad? And that leads us into the whole area of mental illness and detention of the mentally ill. Should we be locking up the mentally ill? We still do it, as discussed in the next chapter.

CHAPTER 4
MAD, BAD OR SAD

There must be a wound! No one can be this hurt and not bleed

– Spike Milligan (Open Heart University).

It was an August Bank Holiday when an elderly lady walked into a large Torquay Hotel. The receptionist could not find her name on the computer but she was insistent.

"I know I'm booked in," she explained, "the Queen booked me in personally." It was then that the receptionist realised that she had a problem. She asked the lady to sit down and rang social services. No, they had not heard of her and, no, they could not help. In desperation, the hotel manager rang the police.

When an officer arrived the elderly lady still insisted that the Queen had booked her in. The hotel appeared to have made a mistake.

After spending time on various phone calls to the health service and social services it became clear no one could help. It was a bank holiday weekend. The Police Officer could not simply send her away; she would not leave and, anyway, where should she go?

Eventually, he took the only course open to him; he took her to the police station under section 136 of the Mental Health Act 1983. If someone appears to a police officer to be suffering from a mental illness, is in a public place and is in need of immediate care and control the officer can take them to a "place of safety." The police station was the only "place of safety" available.

There should have been alternatives. A place of safety can be a specialist hospital, residential accommodation provided by a local social services' authority, a care home for the mentally ill or "any other suitable place ... which is willing temporarily to receive the patient."

When I saw her, she was sitting, still wearing her twin set and pearls, in the "cage"; a large caged-off area which was used to hold detainees waiting to be booked in. It was a Saturday night and various drunks were being brought in, fighting and swearing but she had fewer rights than the drunks. She was detained under the Mental Health Act and not the usual law which oversees custody. Alleged criminals can only be detained for up to twenty four hours before being charged or released. Under the Mental Health Act, she could be detained for up to 72 hours.

I took her to the medical room.

"There appears to have been a bit of a muddle" she said. She had no idea which town she was in or the day of the week. This was clearly not the right place for her but there was nowhere else.

The custody sergeant had found some paperwork in her handbag so we knew her name and we had an address. She was from Notting Hill, West London. He rang her local police and asked whether they knew her? Did she often go on walkabout? What we had forgotten was that this was August Bank Holiday – the weekend of the Notting Hill Carnival. Her local police had larger problems than a little old lady who had turned up in Torquay.

He then rang the local duty social worker who came to see her. Now that she was being detained under the Mental Health Act, social services could no longer claim that it was not their problem. After more research, the social worker found that the address was a residential care home.

He rang the home, who agreed that she was their resident, she was suffering from dementia and, no, she wasn't in her room.

So what had happened? She must have walked out of the home, gone to Paddington Station and got on a train. Somehow she had managed to travel from London to Torquay without ever being asked for a ticket.

It took several hours before social services could arrange transport to get her home; hours in which she sat in a cell in the custody suite. Along with the custody staff and the social worker, I felt angry. Why should we lock an elderly, confused lady in a cell? But then, I had seen too many people with mental health problems ending up in police cells. Have we really moved on from the Victorian days when mental asylums were really prisons?

There was one positive side; we were all agreed what should happen. She needed to go home.

Whenever an officer brought in someone under section 136 "in need of immediate care and control" I always had to call an approved social worker. If the patient needed a mental health assessment, we called the duty psychiatrist or, to use the jargon of the Act, a "section 12 approved doctor". The assessment had to involve two doctors and a social worker. We did not always agree and, if we did agree admission, we frequently found that there was no bed available. This elderly lady with dementia did not need a further assessment.

Another case of dementia was also easy to place. An elderly, slightly confused lady regularly took the same bus into the town for shopping. The bus driver knew her well and understood that she could manage with a little help. Unfortunately one morning the usual bus driver was away. She got on the bus, showed her bus pass but did not appear to know where she was going. This would not have worried the normal driver. He knew where to drop her off but the replacement driver did not know her. When he tried to explain that he could not take her if she did not know where she was going, she became distressed and even more confused. Eventually the police were called and the officer took her to the Police Station, again as a place of safety. Once there, we discovered her name and fortunately managed to contact her daughter, who came and collected her.

Arguments over who should see mentally ill people at a police station are not new. The British Medical Journal in 1884 reported a dispute between the Mayor of Exeter and the local "Medical Men"; presumably there were no medical women in Exeter at the time.

They reported *that "'Till recently the practice of the Police in Exeter in cases of emergency was to call the Police Surgeon. Mr Moon and other surgeons vehemently objected to this (obviously improper) practice and demanded that the nearest medical man should always be sent for"*. The issue then was not the welfare of the patient but the payment for the doctor. In a purely private system the "nearest medical man" was concerned that he was missing a potential fee. But there was another problem; who was to pay this fee?

When the mayor did call a doctor he assumed that they would see the patient for free.

"The Mayor of that city not only thinks that the lunacy laws are imperfect, and that the usual medical certificate is not a conclusive test of sanity or insanity (in which opinion other persons may perhaps agree), but he is apparently impressed with the idea that his position as Mayor entitles him to exercise despotic authority over the medical gentlemen who practise within the area of his jurisdiction. If he think fit, he orders any medical man whom he is pleased to select to examine a patient alleged to be insane; and not only so, but he apparently considers that the holding of such examinations is a part of the public duty which a doctor must perform, for he is reported to have threatened to indict a medical man who refused to examine a patient when bidden, and, on the other hand, to have declined to pay for an examination held by a practitioner whom he had called." Even then it was agreed that the lunacy laws were imperfect. Their successor, the Mental Health Acts 1983 and 1987 still are.

We also had people brought in for a crime who were mentally unwell. Was it their fault? To use the old Latin phrase, the accused has to have *mens rea* or "intention".

Again this is not a new problem. As long ago as 1800 James Hadfield tried to assassinate King George III at the Drury Lane Theatre in London. In court it was argued that he only tried to kill the King because he was suicidal and wanted to get himself killed. The problem faced by the court was that, if he committed the crime due to mental illness they would have to find him not guilty. Most criminals who were judged insane were sent home to their families. But James Hadfield had tried to kill the King. Could he just go home?

The only laws open to the courts were the vagrancy Acts of 1714 and 1744. There were laws dealing with "vagrants" since 1597 but the 1714 Act increased the definition of a vagrant to include "all those who were unable to give a good account of themselves". James Hadfield could not give a good account of himself so he could be detained but under this law but he would have to be released when he "recovered his mind". Might he then have a relapse and try to kill the King again?

After the trial Parliament rapidly passed the Criminal Lunatics Act of 1800. This ruled that anyone acquitted of treason, murder or felony on the grounds of insanity shall still be locked up "at his majesty's pleasure". The courts had to detain the person, mad or not, regardless of the opinion of the judge or jury.

Fortunately, I was never called to see someone who had tried to kill the Queen, even if she had booked them into a Torquay Hotel. However, I was called to cases where the crime was simply a manifestation of a mental illness.

A young man was brought in who had been arrested after attacking his mother. He did not live locally and was angry. He told me that his wife was trying to prove that he was mad but then said "I'm not manic depressive or schizoid."

He was talking continuously, telling me that he worked for a supermarket and used to be in charge of all the hygiene and cleaning

A Police Surgeon's Lot

in the country but had recently had a row with the company over a crack on a tin.

He claimed that he was with the rock band Black Sabbath but was better than their lead guitarist as he was a combination of four rock guitarists. He even named them. He then tried using technical jargon mentioning "demi-semi quavers".

Legally, he told us, he could get out of the police station at any time as he knew all the top barristers and helped them at the Old Bailey.

Physically he was well but, after a few phone calls, we found that he was well known to his local mental health team. Despite his objections, his wife's claims that he suffered from mental illness were true. He was in the manic phase of bipolar disorder.

The assessment from the psychiatrist and social worker confirmed his illness and he was committed under the Mental Health Act. After he had left I tried to sound professional and said to the psychiatrist that he had classic "knight's move thinking, grandiose thoughts and flights of ideas". He smiled and said, "Come on Pete. He's completely bonkers".

Not all cases were so straightforward. Some people are good at hiding the fact that they are completely bonkers.

In March 1996, I was called to Torquay Police Station at half past eleven at night. The custody sergeant told me the history. Sian was 22 and had been arrested for inflicting "actual bodily harm". She had a long psychiatric history and normally lived with her parents in Warwickshire. The family had come down on a short holiday to Devon and were staying about ten miles from Torquay.

Earlier in the evening, she had been in the hotel bar, drinking a low alcohol grape juice when she suddenly hit her father. He was taken to the local Accident and Emergency Department but was not badly hurt.

The custody sergeant had Sian's medication in a 'nomad' box, with separate compartments for each tablet. He also gave me the hotel telephone number.

I rang Sian's mother at the hotel. She had a good understanding of her daughter's illness; she was schizophrenic. She also knew all her medication and the relevant sections of the Mental Health Act 1983. She had even set up and organised a group at her home for parents of schizophrenic patients and so I was dealing with an expert carer.

Sian had been well throughout her childhood but, during her first year as a student at University, she was admitted to a psychiatric hospital suffering from a 'schizo-affective disorder'. She was kept in for a year under a committal, in accordance with the Mental Health Act, which had been renewed regularly. She then returned to University but was still unwell and, eventually, took an overdose. When she had physically recovered, she had been re-admitted to the psychiatric unit and had only been discharged four weeks before the incident.

Her mother was concerned that, recently, she had been deteriorating, although she could not be specific. She wondered whether she was taking her medication. It is a common problem for patients who are well controlled on medication in hospital to refuse their medication when discharged. In the early 1990s there were several high profile cases of patients, who had refused medication, having consequential problems. One of the more notorious was the case of Ben Silcock, a chronic schizophrenic, who climbed into the lion enclosure at London Zoo. Although there are legal ways to ensure patients take their medication, Sian was intelligent and was not going to get caught.

I listened to Sian's mother carefully. She knew her daughter far better than anyone else.

Eventually, I asked her what had happened that night. Apparently, her father had offered her another drink which she then mis-interpreted as a sexual advance.

When I saw Sian she was well dressed and relaxed. She was well spoken and did not appear to be under the influence of alcohol or any other drug.

She told me that she had wanted to study medicine but did not achieve high enough grades at 'A' level. While reading biology, she had been so uncertain and disappointed that she had suffered a 'breakdown'. In the past, she had heard voices in her head which used to keep her awake but she had not had this problem for some time.

When asked about the incident with her father that evening she told me that she was at the bar when her father said: "Do you want one?" She was convinced this was a sexual proposition. When asked why she had interpreted the comment in this way she told me that it was "obvious". She could not accept that there could have been any other explanation for the comment and showed no sign of remorse for the assault. I asked whether her father had ever made any similar advances in the past and she admitted that he had not. She did not believe that she was suffering from a psychiatric problem and did not see the need for hospital admission.

Following my interview, I rang the duty social worker. If needed we could "section" her under the 1983 Mental Health Act. This would mean compulsory admission. Although we still use the word "section" for compulsory admission, this word is not in the Act. Even the definition of mental disorder is a little vague; "Any disorder or disability of mind."

I did not have the power to "section" her; neither did the consultant psychiatrist. In keeping with the prevailing attitude of the 1980s, when the Act was passed, it was not doctors who arrange a section but a social worker. This was widened in 2007 to include some psychiatric nurses but still not doctors. Unfortunately, the social worker was in Plymouth, 30 miles away, although he agreed to attend as soon as he could.

I then rang the duty consultant psychiatrist, who suggested that she be kept in the cells overnight so that we could contact her mental health team in the morning. Legally, she was still there for ABH and so we could keep her in for up to 24 hours.

The social worker agreed to wait until the morning, when we might have a better picture from her local mental health team.

I went through her medication with the duty sergeant, left written instructions and went home to bed at 01.00 am. Since seeing Sian, I had managed to see three other prisoners, between the phone calls.

I did not sleep through. The sergeant rang. Sian's father had withdrawn the complaint. He did not want his daughter locked up for ABH. This was understandable but put us in a difficult position. The only legal power we had to keep her locked up was her alleged offence. Of course, this was only a holding operation. The police had no intention of charging her. In the morning the charges would be dropped once the mental health services were in place. But with the chief witness to the "crime" pulling out, the police had no power to hold her; she should be released forthwith.

The custody sergeant rang Sian's mother. She was very upset, terrified that, if she was released she would kill herself. She had taken an overdose before.

The Sergeant wondered whether we could use the Mental Health Act section 136 - the same power used to bring in the elderly lady with dementia. But this only allows the police to bring someone in from a public place. A police station is not a public place. Could we still hold her for ABH, even though the principle witness had withdrawn his evidence? The only alternative would have been to arrange for the psychiatrist and social worker to carry out an immediate assessment. In the middle of the night, with no notes and without talking to the team who looked after her, this was not ideal. The sergeant said that he would find out and get back to me.

I was delighted when my alarm clock went off in the morning with no further calls. The sergeant must have found a way through the bureaucracy. In hindsight the sergeant could probably have kept her in custody for the ABH as her father is only a witness. Allegations still stand even if a witness pulls out. But the police are, understandably risk averse and do not want to risk being accused of unlawful detention.

Even better news was a message waiting for me from the ward sister of the hospital where Sian had been an in-patient. Her mother had been in touch. Could I ring her?

The message from the ward was "whatever you do, don't release her." She had made several serious attempts at suicide in the past. She was highly intelligent and knew the symptoms of her illness.

To avoid being admitted under the Mental Health Act she would lie about her symptoms. She was 'almost certainly' hearing voices but would only admit this as she improved with treatment. The consultant was willing to send an escort down to Devon to pick her up and admit her to their hospital, provided we agreed to 'section' her under the Mental Health Act.

Our local psychiatrist had been right; we had needed to wait until the morning, to talk to her team.

I saw Sian at 09.20 am. She remembered me and her mental state was unchanged. She still denied hearing voices. I also asked her specifically about any suicidal thoughts and plans. She admitted that, in the past, she had tried to kill herself. However, she remembered her mother's quote from Ben Elton. Every day when he wakes up and tells himself he is glad to be alive. Sian claimed to be following this ideal.

I rang the duty social worker; a different one from the one on duty the previous night. He said that he would attend as soon as possible but he was dealing with a child abuse case ten miles away – fortunately, not one involving the police surgeon.

I then telephoned the duty psychiatrist; again, a different one from the previous night. He suggested that she be assessed by the social worker, before he saw her. Finally, I rang Sian's mother to inform her of our plans.

It was clear that an assessment of Sian, without a discussion with the mental health team who knew her well, might have led to her being released. She was articulate, intelligent and knew the system.

I rang the ward sister again. Could their psychiatrist discuss Sian directly with our local duty psychiatrist?

Although her normal psychiatrist was off duty, he rang me at the police station. He agreed with Sian's mother and the ward sister. Suicide was a high risk. I rang our psychiatrist and gave him his colleague's phone number.

I arranged to meet our local psychiatrist and the social worker at 1pm in the police station.

Sian stuck to her script. She denied any symptoms of mental illness, apart from the rigid belief that her father had been trying to proposition her.

We put it to her that, in view of the real violence she had shown, over a belief which appeared to be unreasonable; the history from her mother, the ward sister and psychiatrist, she would need to be admitted to her local hospital under the Mental Health Act 1983. She accepted the decision commenting that, if two doctors agreed, then she would accept admission. She knew the law.

But did this comment mean that she now agreed to go in to hospital? If it did, then we could not section her. It is only possible to section a patient who is refusing admission.

Luckily, the only person who could authorise the section, the social worker, agreed that this "consent" was only grudgingly made after we had told her that we were admitting her under the Act. Moreover, the escort was to take her on a three hour drive and we could not risk her changing her mind en route.

We decided to rely on section 2 of the 1983 Act. She could be admitted for up to 28 days but only for an assessment. For treatment they would need a section 3 committal, which can last up to six months.

The section 2 committal needed two doctors, one with expertise in psychiatry and one who, ideally, had prior knowledge of the patient. I acted as the second doctor. I did not have prior knowledge of the patient but the situation was not ideal.

The first Madhouse Act, 200 years ago, insisted that assessments could be carried out only by doctors who were members of the Royal College of Physicians but now doctors could only advise admission and not insist. Doctors had been moved from the centre to the periphery and I have seen doctors overruled by social workers in the police station, much to the chagrin of the custody sergeant.

As they left, I wondered whether her reaction had been so unreasonable. Had the mental illness been the result of abuse by her father? Did the question "do you want one" trigger unhappy memories? She was being transferred to a team who knew her well. They are questions which they would ask.

She was clearly at risk but there is a myth that anyone who is mentally ill can be "sectioned". In the custody suite, I have seen angry custody sergeants, after a patient was not sectioned. "But surely he's mad, isn't he doc!" To section a patient it is not just a case of suggesting that they are "mad." The patient has to pose a risk to themselves or others and there must be no viable alternative. If you think you're Napoleon but do not plan to harm yourself or others by creating an Empire or assaulting anyone called Josephine you should be treated in the community.

However, sometimes, people who appear mentally ill are suffering from a physical problem, which his why a doctor or nurse is needed to assess anyone brought into the police station under the Mental Health Act.

Richard Watt was in his thirties had no history of mental health problems. He was married with a family, had a job and was living in a typical three bedroom semi-detached house. One day, he started behaving strangely. He went to his neighbours carrying a clip board and told them that they were on "This is your life". For those of you too young to remember the programme, it ran through the biography of a celebrity, reintroducing him to various people from the past. But these neighbours were not celebrities and he was not working for the television company. The police were called and he was taken to the police station under section 136. When I saw him, he was unwell with a high temperature. His chest showed signs of acute lobar pneumonia. I admitted him to hospital, where he was treated and recovered. There was no mental illness but an acute confusional state from pneumonia.

In another case, a man walked into a gentleman's club, claiming to own the building. He again was detained under section 136 and, again, was clearly very unwell. I admitted him into the acute medical ward, although I had no idea of the diagnosis. I spoke to the medical registrar as I knew that a junior house officer might refuse "an obvious psychiatric case".

After a battery of tests, the medical team found a high salicylate level. He had come to Paignton to commit suicide, booked into a guest house and taken an overdose of aspirin. Instead of killing him, the overdose made him confused and he left the guest house for the club.

So underlying that physical problem, was a possible mental illness;which brings us back to the debate whether someone who decides to kill himself is mentally ill or has made a rational decision. After time in the intensive care unit, he survived. If he had taken paracetamol instead, I would probably have seen him as a body found in the guest house.

I also experienced another side; people who were not mentally or physically unwell but who tried to use feigned mental illness as a 'get out of jail free' card.

Sharon was a regular in custody. She was a prolific burglar and shoplifter but, whenever arrested, she played the mental health card; trying to argue that the crimes were not her fault. She was mentally ill. She had seen the mental health team and been assessed several times by psychiatrists. There was no evidence of any mental illness. She knew exactly what she was doing and had been told that she must take responsibility for her own behaviour. Unfortunately, there had been one occasion when a psychiatrist had made a passing comment about borderline personality disorder and so, every time she was arrested, she claimed that she did not know what she was doing. The night in question when I saw her, I happened to be working with a consultant psychiatrist seeing another patient. When we had finished, the custody sergeant asked me to assess Sharon's mental health. The duty psychiatrist knew her and knew her modus operandi. We saw her together and spent time assessing her mental state. We both wrote a statement saying that there was no evidence of mental illness and that she must take responsibility for her actions.

A few days later, I asked the sergeant whether he knew the court's verdict. Yes. Both statements were read out, but her solicitor insisted that the alleged crime was a result of her mental condition.

She could not help her behaviour. The magistrate referred her for a mental health assessment, before sentence. Courts are aware of the large number of people, with mental health problems, in prison and do not want to make the situation worse. Some judges and magistrates cannot ignore any suggestion of a mental health problem from the defence, however manipulative.

To be convicted of most serious criminal offences the offender has to be proved to show "mens rea" or a guilty intention. If someone is seriously mentally unwell and the illness leads to an ostensible crime, should they be punished? If, for example, a schizophrenic hears voices telling him that the person standing by him is the devil and to attack, he would honestly believe he was helping the world in launching the attack. He would not have mens rea.

When working in prisons I saw several people, like Sharon, who claimed they could not help committing the crime, blaming a mental illness. They hid behind a psychiatric label, failing to accept responsibility for their own actions. This is not the same as those with a genuine mental illness. Some inmates claimed their crime was not their fault, although they had had several thorough assessments by several psychiatrists, all of whom found no mental illness. However, it can be difficult to assess whether someone is genuinely mentally unwell. After all, if someone tells me they are hearing voices, I can't do a blood test or x-ray to check.

In 2012 I was involved in setting up a liaison and diversion scheme. Logically, we needed to divert prisoners with mental health problems out of the criminal justice system altogether and into healthcare. As far back as 1990, the Bradley report had pointed out that community punishments are more effective than prison for people with mental health problems.

It had been estimated that ninety per cent. of people in prison have a mental illness and they all come through police custody. Should we be picking these problems up before they reach court?

In prisons, ten per cent of inmates suffer from depression; three point seven per cent have a psychotic illness (such as schizophrenia or bipolar disorder) and sixty five per cent have a personality disorder. A large number also have a history of drug and substance abuse. Some of these people may have developed their illness in prison but could we have picked up any in custody?

We now have a liaison and diversion scheme when mental health workers are based in police stations and can called to assess a prisoner's mental state. They have access to the mental health records and can "divert" the patient to the mental health services. However, the question that challenges everyone is when should someone with a mental illness be "diverted?"

Ideally, if the police are called to an incident where the perpetrator appears to be mentally unwell they should be able to call in mental health services straight away. However diversion is more likely to take place in custody, when a forensic nurse or doctor sees the detained person.

How to help a patient in the police station who was mentally ill had been a problem in Exeter in 1884 and one hundred years later, for an elderly lady in Torquay, who thought the Queen had booked her into a hotel. It is not surprising that I did not solve the problem during my time as a "hands-on" FME.

CHAPTER 5
NOT LIKE SEX AT ALL

Rape is not like incompetent or bad sex; it is not like sex at all.

(anon victim)

Life had not been easy for Mandy, a woman in her mid twenties who lived alone in a flat. Her parents had broken up when she was young. Her childhood boyfriend did not want her to go to college, so she stayed with him and worked locally but this was not enough. Whenever she wanted to go out on her own, he would slap her around the face. As the violence increased she realised he wanted to control her. She was "his property".

She moved to Torquay to escape and had landed a good job. She was now working to gain more qualifications. She was still on the pill but no longer had a regular partner.

After work one Friday evening, she went for a drink with Kelvin, a work colleague. They met a group of friends. She could not remember how much she drank but remembered starting with double vodkas and moving on to 'alcopops'

When the pubs shut, she asked him back to her flat for coffee. It was late and raining; he had missed the last bus and had no money for a taxi. She agreed that he could sleep on the settee in the lounge when she went on to bed.

She woke at about 04.00 am to find Kelvin on top of her. Her nightdress had been removed and he had penetrated her. She pushed at his chest, in an attempt to get him off. He then grabbed her forearms and pinned them on either side of her head. His grip was painful and she could not move her upper body. She struggled, trying to get her arms free. He lost his grip three or four times but was on top of her for about ten minutes. She was unsure whether he ejaculated. Later on, she remembered that he bit her breasts once or twice but not hard enough to break the skin.

The following day, she was extremely sore and noticed a number of small bruises to both her upper arms and a larger bruise to her left shin. Slowly, she started to remember.

On the Sunday she went to the Police.

She was allocated to Liz, a Sexual Offence Liaison Officer or SOLO. Liz was specially trained to develop a relationship with the victim and help her through the process. She would also keep in touch, throughout investigation, helping Mandy to understand how the case was proceeding and ensuring that she had appropriate follow up.

But it was also vital that we all remember to keep an open mind. False allegations of a sexual offence can devastate a man's life. Even if he is shown to be innocent there is a danger that others may argue that there is "no smoke without fire." If convicted he will probably lose his job and could lose his family. Everyone is innocent until proven guilty.

Mandy's case took place in the 1990s. I saw her in the local sexual assault suite when I was also on call for all the other police work. These suites were a huge improvement on the previous examinations in a police station medical room but still had problems. Care for victims and the collection of evidence was often patchy. Most of the doctors were male. These suites were still run by the police, which did not help victims, who were already afraid to report a rape or sexual assault.

Within the suite, was a fully equipped medical examination room as well as facilities for making tea and coffee and a shower for the victim after the examination. She could, though, have been kept waiting or I could have received other calls during the examination. Sometimes, rape victims even complained that the examination felt like another violation.

Liz had already sat with Mandy in the lounge and taken a detailed history using the "Blue book", a long proforma ensuring that she asked all the relevant questions.

When I arrived I had a quiet word with Liz so that I knew the allegations. I needed some idea, so that I could target the examination. I did not want Mandy to have to go through all the details again. She had had enough. Luckily I had worked with Liz several times before and we got on well.

I tried to be as understanding as possible; sitting and listening. I sat down with her in the lounge and explained that I was a GP, with some extra training, to help in these difficult situations. I found this approach less threatening than calling myself a forensic medical examiner or even police surgeon. The GP "bedside manner" is vital. Such an examination must not feel like a second assault. I also needed to ensure that she understood the consent form that she had signed, agreeing to the examination. The examination also had to follow normal practice. A defence lawyer might pick up any deviation.

Mandy was calm and I noted her general state. She was not drunk and did not appear to be under the influence of any other drug. This may have been obvious on a Sunday morning but I had to be prepared for any allegation made by a defence lawyer in court.

I carefully noted the bruises on her arms and legs and drew them onto a body chart. There were no other injuries on the rest of her body.

I took samples of her hair and cut her fingernails and more intimate samples, all the time ensuring that she was covered when possible. Today we would use a colposcope and take intimate photographs but this was not available in the 1990s. She was uninjured around the vagina, although this did not exclude her having been raped. If her allegations were true, there was no reason why she should be injured.

A few weeks later, I heard that the swabs did not show any semen. A positive result would have proved that they had had sex but a negative result did not prove anything. A man does not need to ejaculate to be guilty of rape; although this was the case until 1828.

The popular image of rape is of a psychopath leaping out from the hedge and jumping on a passing woman; indeed the old common law definition was "ravished against the King's peace." However, for almost two hundred years, rape has simply meant sexual intercourse without consent. In the nineteenth century, the common law used the words *"carnal knowledge of a woman and against her will"*. The idea that, somehow, the Victorians were misogynistic and did not care is unfair. Until 1841, conviction of rape carried the death penalty.

As recently as 1976, an Old Bailey Judge, HHJ Edward Sutcliffe QC, said to jury in a rape case *"it is well known that women in particular and small boys are liable to be untruthful and invent stories"*, suggesting that, in some quarters, sexual assault and rape were still not understood.

In Mandy's case, the court had to decide whether Mandy and Kelvin had had sex and, if they had, had Mandy agreed to it? Both sides agreed that they had had sex. The argument was over consent. But what does "consent" mean? A loving couple, who have been married for twenty years, do not have, or need, a pile of consent forms by the bed.

The case occurred in the 1990s, when I was working under the rules of the old Sexual Offences Act 1956. All the court needed to ask was would a "reasonable man" have assumed she agreed? This explains why, in the past, barristers would ask victims what they were wearing and suggest that their behaviour had been provocative. If a girl takes a man back to her flat, strips off and goes to bed, smiles and says "you wouldn't, would you" would a "reasonable man" assume that she had agreed to sex? By taking her back to her flat, was it reasonable for Kelvin to believe that she had agreed to have sex? Under this old law it did not matter whether the victim did not consent provided "a reasonable man" would have interpreted her behaviour as saying 'yes'.

Kelvin was arrested and charged with rape. The Magistrates' Court committed him for trial at the Crown Court. He was remanded in custody but, later, released on bail, on the condition that he stayed with his mother and did not attempt to communicate with Mandy.

In court I could not say exactly when the bruises were inflicted. I agreed that there were no other injuries. The defence argued that she consented to sex. She did invite him back to her flat. Would a "reasonable man" have assumed this was consent?

After six hours of deliberation, the jury returned a unanimous verdict of not guilty. I had seen her distress but only heard one side of the story. I had not heard all the evidence. If she had really been asleep it is hard to see how the jury could have decided that she consented to sex. Did they hear an alternative explanation for the bruises? If there was any doubt about whether she was asleep, whether her version of events was accurate then the jury had to acquit Kelvin. There would have been "reasonable doubt".

A new Sexual Offences Act was passed in 2003. This new law has a much tighter definition of consent. Now the court has to ask: "What did the man do to ensure she agreed?" At last, the law accepted that saying 'no' means no, however she behaved. The onus is now on the man to explain what he did to ensure she was consenting.

Although common for victims of any crime, rape is far more likely to lead to mental health problems, in the victim; especially in the common situation when the victim already knows the assailant.

I have seen a large number of victims of alleged sexual abuse or rape. It was not over after they leave the court.

When asked about stress, most people think of the classic post-traumatic stress disorder but this is only one of a number of mental health problems that can result from stress. More common than PTSD is substance misuse, often seen in ex- servicemen. The tragedy for these people is that while the symptoms of PTSD in an ex-serviceman or woman produces sympathy, the alcohol or drug abuse to which they then resort, may produce derision. Substance abuse is still seen as self-inflicted.

Stress may lead to long-term depression and panic attacks. The victims feel helpless.

Rape is not the same as other trauma. Rape is about as personal as it gets. A tsunami, earthquake or shipping disaster is not personal. If the victim knew and trusted the assailant, she will question the motivation of everyone. She may have had feelings towards the assailant; such feelings have not just gone and she may still have to see him around, at home, at work, in the street and she will still be frightened. How can someone in Mandy's position go back to work if the acquitted defendant is also there?

Mandy also had to face the fact that the jury believed, essentially, that she was lying. Rape is still seen as "ravished against the King's peace." I did not hear all the evidence in Mandy's case and the jury felt that the prosecution could not prove beyond reasonable doubt that she did not consent to sex.

In the popular press rape means a stranger jumping out from behind a bush, not a work colleague invited back. Even if Kelvin had been found guilty and it had been shown that Mandy did not consent to sex, in the eyes of many people this would not be "real rape".

Rape victims feel self-doubt; did she encourage him? Did she send out the wrong message? She feels guilty and dirty. Cross examination from the defence lawyer can add extra trauma but it may be the only way to avoid wrongful conviction. .

When the allegation is not rape but "sexual assault", to a victim, there is nothing sexual about it; it is an assault, usually through fear and domination. It is not incompetent or bad sex; it is not like sex at all.

Fortunately, the whole management of rape and sexual assault has now changed. Trace evidence is vital but so is a sensitive handling of the victim.

In 1986 a Sexual Assault Referral Centre (SARC) was set up in Manchester. This was based in a woman's hospital, St Mary's and provided a "one stop shop." Anyone arriving at the centre was met by a crisis worker, who explained the process and obtained consent to examination. On the same site, victims were offered forensic and medical examinations, one-to-one counselling, screening for sexually transmitted diseases, pregnancy testing and post-coital contraception or the "morning after pill." There was also 24-hour phone support.

The SARC concept has now been rolled out nationally. Many are run by charities with the police and medical team as "guests."

Although the examination has never been pleasant for the victim, careful handling can make it more bearable.

A local girls' boarding school employed an odd-job man but, after a few weeks, he was dismissed. I was not told why. One night the following week the residential matron was sexually assaulted in the night. She woke up to find the man on top of her. He admitted burglary but claimed that he did not go near her. She had been asleep and was unclear what had happened.

As I examined her, I was chatting. It turned out that she had been a student nurse in London at the same time that I had been a student; we had been at rival hospitals. As she relaxed, she suddenly remembered something she had not told the police. "I think he licked my breast just here, I'm not sure." I took a swab and, a few weeks later, I received a delighted phone call from the officer involved. "We got a DNA hit, doc." His defence that he had not gone near her fell apart and he was sent to prison for eight years

After the case, I received a letter from the victim. My approach had "made an unbearable experience more bearable." Chatting about issues that appear irrelevant could be vital provided I did not discuss any issue, which might have tended to alter her memory. As well as physical contamination it was possible to "contaminate" her memory of events. In court the barrister might argue "did this really happen or did the doctor put this idea in your mind?"

Several other changes occurred in the early 2000s. The sexual offences' work was separated from custody work, reducing the risk of contamination. A doctor called from a custody centre may inadvertently pick up trace evidence from a detainee who has nothing to do with the case, risking contamination of the samples. It was also hoped that most of the doctors who examine victims of sexual assault should be women who specialise in this work. All victims are given a choice of a male or female doctor but this is not always practicable. Recruitment is a problem.

The expertise of the doctor may be more important than the gender. A very experienced male colleague of mine was asked to see a victim who really wanted a female doctor. Working with my colleague was a young female GP trainee. She was a fully qualified doctor, who had worked in a gynaecology department but had no experience in forensic work. My colleague agreed to let her do the examination. He would wait outside and be available for any help or advice.

The examination went well. Her examination and samples were ideal, until the court case. Although he could not find fault with her examination, sample-taking or notes, the defence barrister realised what had happened.

"So, how much training have you had for this highly specialised work?"

"How many cases have you done before today?"

He pointed out to the jury that she had no training or experience and then asked "how can we accept this evidence beyond reasonable doubt when the doctor had no training and no experience?" This was a fair point. A detailed forensic examination requires specialist training. The accused was acquitted and a lesson was learnt. Training and experience are more important than the doctor's gender although a victim should always be given the choice provided the male and female doctors are equally competent.

Separating custody work from sexual offences' work also removed a problem. Anyone who has had any contact with the alleged offender must not go near the alleged victim; otherwise the court will argue that his DNA is only on her because of cross contamination. In theory, the same doctor may examine the alleged victim and the alleged offender but only if he or she goes home, has a shower and changes all their clothes. In one case, I was called out to another area, to examine a suspect, because the local duty doctor had examined the victim. This sounded reasonable. It was only when I arrived that I discovered that his examination of the victim had taken place six months before. When I met him at a meeting I did express concern that the Police obviously thought that he had not washed or changed his clothes for six months.

There is another issue. Both the alleged victim and defendant might have been drinking. In 2014, a retired Judge, H.H. Mary Mowat, suggested that we would not improve rape conviction rates unless women cut their drinking. She suggested that, if someone was "off their head" and couldn't remember anything, but wakes up the next day feeling sore and makes allegations how should a jury react?

In 2005, in a case at Swansea Crown Court when a security guard was accused of raping a student who was too drunk to remember whether she agreed to have sex Judge Roderick Evans ruled that drunken consent is still consent. But in 2007 (R vs Bree) the Court of Appeal ruled that if a woman had temporally lost her capacity to choose to have sex it is rape. However if she had consumed a large quantity of alcohol but still had the capacity to choose it is not rape. The question arises if the alleged victim is very drunk, does she have the capacity to agree to sex? After all, if someone signs a legal document, when very drunk, it could be challenged. Moreover, if an alleged perpetrator buys a woman alcohol purely to get her drunk and reduce her capacity say 'no', then it would be rape. The challenge would be to prove his motive "beyond reasonable doubt" in court.

Alleged victims may not deliberately lie but alcohol metabolism differs between men and women. In the "ladette" culture, many girls simply do not realise how much they have drunk. One director of a sexual assault referral centre, in a city centre, near a red light district, told me that local prostitutes complain that some men found it easier and cheaper to have sex with drunk girls leaving clubs than paying for the "service."

It was a part of the routine assessment of an alleged victim of sexual assault to test for drugs. Did the offender spike her drink? It was very rare for any of these tests to show anything apart from alcohol. This could be because the other drugs had worn off and were now undetectable but a part of the routine was to take a urine sample, as soon as possible, rather than wait for the full medical examination. Nothing justifies rape and other sexual assaults. Women should be just as free as men to get drunk but the idea that drinks are often spiked with date-rape drugs does not fit with my experience.

I once saw a young girl who believed that her drink has been spiked. She told me that she had not drunk very much. When I asked her how much, she said, "Only about twelve Jack Daniels". Blood samples found only alcohol.

In June 2004 a report in our local paper, quoted an alleged rape victim and read: *I was in a pub in Paignton and briefly put my drink on the bar. About 15 minutes after taking a sip I was violently sick and could not stand up*".

Think about this case. Even if her drink was a single short, it would still be at least 25 mls. One sip would be 5 mls at the most. She could only have had twenty per cent. of the drink at most and, probably, far less. For most date-rape drugs, the effective dose is usually two tablets, crushed into powder. This means that the offender would have to have slipped in at least ten tablets to have given her a normal dose, from one sip. To cause such severe drowsiness she would probably need about ten times the normal dose. Is it possible that someone slipped in a hundred tablets without her noticing and without it affecting the taste and colour of the drink? I'm sorry but I think that she was already very drunk when she took her sip.

In 2006 the Association of Chief Police Officers (ACPO) conducted "Operation Matisse". They looked at one hundred and twenty cases of use of alleged "date-rape" drugs for a year from: London, Manchester, Walsall, Derbyshire, Northumbria and Lancashire. Only one of the one hundred and twenty victims had not been drinking alcohol. Twenty-two of the girls had blood alcohol levels nearly three times the drink-drive limit.

Another study, in Northern Ireland, found similar results, with the average blood alcohol level of victims being 217 mgs in 100 mls of blood compared to the drink-drive limit of 80 mgs in 100 mls of blood. Over 200 mgs is very drunk. Research in Australia also came to the conclusion that "many individuals consumed large volumes of alcohol prior to the alleged assault."

Over the years, it was standard practice to test the drug levels of victims; not to make a judgement but in case we were dealing with a "date rape" drug. The term "date rape" was coined by Karen Barrett, in September 1982, in an article in Ms Magazine, entitled "Date rape: a campus epidemic?" Forensically, we use the more accurate - – but less catchy title - – "drug facilitated sexual assault" or DFSA.

Although there are plenty of anecdotal stories of rohypnol and other drugs being used to facilitate sexual assault, in thirty years of dealing with sexual assaults, I have found that these cases are rare. The usual "date- rape" drug is alcohol.

Reading the popular press, it appears that the crime of drugging a woman before rape is not now only common but a new problem. It is neither.

In 1855 the British Medical Journal said, *"There are many instances on record of stupefying drugs having been employed for the purpose of facilitating the perpetration of the crime of rape ... and the fact that their victim was unconscious does not in the smallest degree lessen the criminality of the deed"*.

They reported a case, in December 1854, from Philadelphia. *"A young lady, of unimpeachable character, who had for some time been engaged to be married, was accompanied by her betrothed to the house of an ancient and highly respectable dentist"*. She alleged that, after being put to sleep with ether she had a *"distinct memory"* that he *"put his hand on my arm under my sleeve; ....he put his hand on my breast, under my dress; on the bosom; he put his hand on my person, under my dress"*. I do not need to clarify the word "person". But the situation got worse. She went on to claim that, *"he drew me down to the edge of the chair; I do not know what he did after that till I felt pain; he did enter my person; it was then I felt the pain"*. Although she was not examined, as she was menstruating, the dentist was convicted.

The BMJ did not agree, arguing that: *"The only direct and positive testimony was that of the young lady herself"* Apparently ether *"does tend to excite the erotic propensities"*, which makes it sound like an ideal drug for a rapist to give to a victim. But the BMJ argued that the situation was made worse on the *"hyper-sensitive frame of an American lady"*. A modern, forensic physician might have a problem finding evidence that American ladies have hypersensitive frames.

The one strong argument with which we would all accept is that *"No medical man should administer an anaesthetic to females without a third party being present."* Today, we would advise the presence of a chaperone at any examination of a female by a "medical man".

Nearly a hundred and fifty years after the BMJ article, the 2003 Act contained very similar phraseology. There is no consent to intercourse if the woman is *"stupefied or overpowered by substance administered without consent."* So it is rape if the woman is "out of it" after being given a drug and are date rape drugs common or an urban myth?

In Operation Matisse, nearly half the alleged victims had other drugs in their system but the commonest drugs were cannabis and cocaine. Cannabis is usually smoked and cocaine is a stimulant so neither could be used as a covert, sedative "date-rape" drug. There were no cases of the famous "Rohypnol", the drug quoted in the popular press as being at the forefront of "date rape" drugs. There were only ten cases of Gamma Hydroxybutyric Acid (GHB) the other likely candidate.

Another large study, in the UK, by the Forensic Science in London surveyed over one thousand urine and blood tests, of alleged victims, in cases of alleged DFSA. In thirty five per cent of cases, there was no drug at all found. Of the cases in which drugs were detected, thirty one per cent showed only alcohol and forty six per cent showed alcohol with an illicit drug. Nineteen per cent showed only an illicit drug.

So, what drugs were detected? Not all the drugs could have been administered illicitly by an alleged rapist.

One in four was positive for cannabis. This is usually smoked but, even if taken by mouth, it is unlikely it would be slipped into a drink and it is very slow-acting orally.

Eleven per cent were positive for cocaine. This is a stimulant and so unlikely to dull the mind. It might give the victim a feel-good factor but would this be enough for her to consent to sex when she would otherwise refuse?

Ecstasy which has the full chemical name of methylenedioxymethamphetamine (MDMA) was present in five per cent of cases and other amphetamines were present in in two per cent. Again, these are stimulants and the same argument applies as would apply for cocaine.

One in a hundred alleged victims had heroin, usually given by injection or smoking. It is inactive orally and so is unlikely to have been given surreptitiously, to facilitate a sexual assault.

A half a per cent of cases showed ketamine; again, an unlikely candidate as a "date rape" drug. There was no rohypnol found. So my own experience of similar cases was echoed by this evidence.

I recall the case of a man in his fifties, who was brought in by the police, after complaints that he had been driving through the town with his penis exposed. I only saw him to assess whether he was mentally fit to interview.

As this was before the 2003 Act he was charged under the Vagrancy Act of 1834. In this Act indecent exposure was defined as *"Every person wilfully and obscenely exposing his person in any street, road, or public highway, or in the view thereof, or in any place of public resort with intent to insult any female, may be apprehended and dealt with as a rogue and vagabond"*. The definition of his "person" has been defined in case law and means the penis although this is not the word most men use today. .

If he had only exposed himself because he had been desperate to run to the nearest toilet, it would not be indecent exposure. This was unlikely. The evidence was that he had "intent to insult a female."

Although there are nudist beaches in Devon, I have never seen an arrest under the same statute, which also states *"Men who bathe without any screen or covering near to a public footpath that exposure of their persons must necessarily occur"* are guilty of an indictable nuisance. It is interesting to see that naked women were not considered a nuisance, probably because all law makers in 1834 were men.

Sometimes, to get a conviction, the prosecution had to compromise.

I remember a fifteen-year-old victim called Georgina, known to all as Georgie, who I saw with a female consultant paediatrician in a specially adapted area in the local hospital. I knew the paediatrician well as I had worked with her and we even organised a course on child protection together. To avoid too much trauma to Georgie, we agreed that I should take the lead, although we would both make our own records. Two doctors firing questions and examining her might have added to her distress.

Before even seeing Georgie we took a history from her mother, who told us what Georgie had told her. Legally this is hearsay, but this was not the history to be used in court. It simply helped us understand the allegations. Interviewing a child for court is a specialist job, and if we had asked her directly the defence could argue that we "put ideas in to her head". We also needed to see her mother to obtain written consent for the examination.

She was playing in a lane near her home when she saw Wayne in his back garden. He was in his forties and a family friend. He suggested they meet in five minutes at the bottom of the road to go to the local shops. She agreed; after all he was not a stranger but a family friend. Instead of heading to the shops he drove to a nearby country park.

She remembered his comment "this is enough out of the way" and after talking for a while he suggested that they go in the back of the van. She agreed. It was a cold January and might be warmer. Once in the back he put a foam mattress on the floor and pushed her down on her back. She was scared. He pulled her trousers and pants down, undid his zip and had intercourse with her. She was unsure whether he had ejaculated but noticed sperm on the mattress when she got dressed.

The next day her teacher noticed that she was distressed. When she sat down to talk she told the teacher everything. The teacher contacted social services, who then told the police.

A female officer had taken a good history from Georgie, and we were informed that she hadn't even had her first period yet.

She was a young, brave, woman who coped with the examination well. She was wearing the clothes she had been wearing at the time of the assault, so these were taken and sent to the forensic lab, along with all the swabs to examine for any evidence that might have been left on the body or the clothes.

Four days later, Wayne was arrested on suspicion of rape. He was interviewed at Torquay police station where he vehemently denied the allegations. My colleague took blood for DNA and grouping, hair and saliva samples. He was then released on police bail.

A Police Surgeon's Lot

Nothing was found on her vaginal swabs, but the lab found that her underpants were heavily stained with semen. The forensic scientist concluded that the presence of semen "very strongly supported the assertion" that these pants were worn after an act of sexual intercourse.

But proving it was Wayne's DNA was not so easy. He had had a vasectomy so that there were no sperm cells in his semen. No cells in the 1990s made checking for DNA difficult. However there was a chance. A new technique called Short Tandem Repeat (S.T.R.) had recently been developed. The labs could now take a very small piece of DNA. By repeated cycles of heating and cooling they had discovered that it would replicate more DNA. A minute fraction could become a fraction large enough to test. This was tried on both the semen from the pants and on the accused's blood. The DNA matched. We had evidence of sexual activity "beyond reasonable doubt".

Georgie was so distressed that, several months later, she took an overdose and was admitted to hospital. Although her life was never at risk, it was felt that she would not be able to give evidence in court without it causing her severe distress. It would be impossible to prove rape beyond reasonable doubt without her evidence and so the charge was reduced to unlawful sexual intercourse, on the grounds that intercourse had taken place when the girl was under sixteen.

Although Georgie was clear that she did not consent, without her evidence in court this would have been difficult to prove beyond reasonable doubt. The prosecution had the choice. They could have charged him with rape with a real possibility that he would be acquitted, or accept his guilty plea of unlawful sexual intercourse. At least he would end up with a past conviction and be put on the sexual offender's register. It was not ideal but may help protect others in future. This was in the mid nineteen nineties. In 1999 the Youth Justice and Criminal Evidence Act allowed special measures so that children such as Georgie could give evidence by a link to the court or by video. This might have changed the outcome.

One summer we had a series of stranger-rapes in Devon and Cornwall. I examined some of the victims. We had a detailed description and his DNA. The police had made progress until the body of a man was found hanging in the South East of England. He had committed suicide. His DNA and description matched the rapist. This may have been remorse but, more likely, he knew an arrest was imminent. It is likely that he would have been convicted but, statistically, we had a series of serious stranger- rapes that joined the statistics as "unsolved".

So far I have only discussed the problems of the victims; the law, the dangers of alcohol and drugs and the mental trauma. It has almost become unacceptable to suggest that false accusations even exist. But we do not want to return to the days when some cases alleged victims were not taken seriously, adding to the trauma.

Over the years I have dealt with many cases of sexual assault. They are all unpleasant and traumatic for all concerned. At first sight this appeared to be one of the worst cases I had seen.

I was called out, in the middle of the night, to examine Miss J. She was clearly distressed but had managed to give a short statement to the police. Although she had had a few drinks she was not drunk and did not appear to be under the influence of any other drugs. She had been clubbing in Torquay and, during the evening, a man had approached her but she made it clear that she was not interested. For the rest of the evening he had been watching her. She found him scary.

She left the club on the harbour side in Torquay at about midnight and walked up the main road, alone. She then realised that he was following her. When she turned off into a side street, he ran up to her, pushed her against a wall and raped her.

When I examined her, she had grazes over her buttocks and there was evidence of recent sexual intercourse. I was told that a man had been arrested.

I wrote up my notes, sorted out all the samples and finally went back home to see whether I could salvage some sleep. Detailed notes were vital. This was a case, which was almost certain to end in court.

The following day, I received a phone call from the senior investigating officer. I thought he'd be ringing to ask for a statement. Instead he said, "You know the case you dealt with last night?" How could I forget? "Well, we've looked at the CCTV footage. She left the club with the alleged offender with their arms around each other and kissing".

Of course, that is not consent to intercourse and so we could have still been dealing with a rape but we showed her the CCTV. She admitted that the sex was consensual. When she got home her boyfriend started asking questions and so, rather than admit that she was unfaithful, she claimed she had been raped.

To save her relationship she had put at risk the liberty and reputation of an innocent man. He could have spent eight years in prison and spent his life on the sexual offender's register. Did she really believe that her reputation and relationship with her boyfriend justified ruining someone else's life. Perhaps she just did not think it through.

This was followed by another case which clearly first appeared to be a false allegation. A woman was walking in the countryside, when a stranger pushed her over by a farm gate and raped her. This sounded like the old definition of "ravished against the King's peace." She appeared relaxed and there were no marks anywhere. I took swabs but, again, there was no obvious semen or other evidence. I even visited the scene with the senior officer. The gateway was covered in sharp stones and so we agreed that it was impossible to be pushed onto this surface, have had her pants forcibly removed and have been raped without there being any marks.

However, DNA was found on my samples that matched a known offender. He was arrested and admitted the crime, giving the same details as the victim.

Clinical forensic medicine was never straightforward and both victims and accused needed to be treated with compassion. However, it is not the doctor's job to make judgements, but just to collect the medical evidence and present it in the most neutral manner.

CHAPTER 6
I'LL DRIVE; I'M TOO DRUNK TO SING.

"If you drink and drive you're a bloody idiot."

Australian drink/drive campaign.

Driving when drunk was an offence long before I started as a police surgeon. The law surrounding drinking and driving even pre-dates the motorcar.

Under the Licensing Act 1872 it became an offence to be drunk in charge of cattle, a horse, a carriage or a steam engine. The punishment was a fine up to 40 shillings (£2) or imprisonment, which could include hard labour, for up to one month.

In 1897 George Smith, a 25 year old London taxi driver, was the first person to be arrested for driving a motor vehicle while drunk. He slammed his cab into a building, pleaded guilty and was fined 25 s (£1.25). Even when I started as a police surgeon in the 1970s, attitudes had not changed since Barbara Castle, as Minister of Transport, had brought in the breathalyser in 1967. I saw men, and it usually was men, brought in for drink-driving shouting at the police "why aren't you out catching the real criminals?" Drink-drivers were often wealthy and middle class while burglars were usually poor, deprived and often drug addicts.

By the mid 1960s, the evidence was overwhelming. Research, using driving simulators, showed that driving is affected however much alcohol there is in the blood, so any amount of drink will make a difference to how people drive. Even when the blood level is less than 20 mgs there is increased drowsiness and inattention, and that inattention could kill a child. Between 20 and 50mgs, judgement and vision are affected. At 40 mgs, half the current English legal limit, all measurements of driving skills are impaired.

In some ways the evidence linking alcohol and road accidents followed a similar pattern to the link between smoking and lung cancer. Like smoking and cancer, the effect of drink on driving was medically clear but ignored for a long time; no one wanted to hear

The breathalyser law in 1967 was passed in the face of strong opposition in Parliament, from the motoring organizations and from the publicans. It was seen as an attack on civil liberties. Barbara Castle became a figure of hate and even received death threats. The 1960s was a time when sexism was prevalent and the fact that she was a woman who did not drive made the uproar even more intense. One politician even pointed out that not only did Barbara Castle not drive but, even worse, *"how can a woman possibly understand anything about driving."* I do not know how my mother reacted to these comments. She drove lorries during the second world war and had to maintain and service her own vehicles.

The police were concerned that stopping drivers who might have been drinking would damage public relations and so it was agreed that the police could stop drivers only if they were committing other offences such as speeding.

The breathalyser was only a screening test. If positive, the driver was taken to the police station for a blood or urine test. If the alcohol level was above 80 mgs they were charged. It did not matter if the driver appeared sober; the crime was simply driving with an alcohol level above 80 mgs. Very soon Barbara Castle was proved right. In the first year of the new Act, there were 1,152 fewer fatalities, 11,177 fewer serious injuries and 28,130 fewer slight injuries.

The Police still do not have the power to stop drivers at random but they do stop anyone driving erratically, which includes most of us at some time.

I was once stopped driving home from the Police Station in the middle of the night. I suspect I was driving erratically. I was tired. Once the officers saw me they apologised and continued to apologise when I was next at the Police Station. I did not mind; if I had been a drunk driver I would have been putting other people's lives at risk.

In the 1970s we relied on the 1967 Act which simply stated that it was an offence for anyone with an alcohol level above 80 mgs/100 mls of blood to be "in charge" of a motor vehicle. "In charge" did not necessarily mean driving; just sitting in the driving seat with the keys was enough.

Even today there is an attitude that driving under the influence of alcohol is not really a crime. If I google "drink-drive" a list of companies and solicitors appears offering to help. "Have you been caught drink-driving?" If I google "burglary" there is no similar list of law firms. Is drink driving not really serious, an offence which does not matter unless you're caught, or is it that offenders have more money and are often more respectable?

I was once the target of one drink-driver's anger when taking a sample. He was very drunk, pointed at me and shouted to the police "look at him, he's been drinking, or is on something." He then decided that my tourniquet was dirty and unhygienic. I even got the police photographer to take a picture of my tourniquet. It was clean.

I used the non-alcohol skin wipes although the amount of alcohol on a normal surgical spirit wipe would be so little that it would not affect the result. But I knew that there had been a problem in Manchester when several people accused of drinking and driving had their charges dropped when it was discovered that the doctors were using the wrong swabs.

I also used an old fashioned needle and syringe although in my surgery blood was taken using a vacutainer; a vacuum tube we simply push onto the end of the needle. It is easier, quicker and safer The law states that one sample of blood must be taken and split into two, one of which is given to the accused to have analysed at their own expense. Of course using a vacutainer and filling two bottles would be as accurate but, legally, it is not one sample but two.

Inside I was seething. This arrogant man was accusing me of a serious breach of ethics. He was the one putting other people's lives at risk by drink-driving. I would never go to work drunk or on any other drug. I managed to maintain my professional veneer; not even commenting on his offensive accusations. But perhaps my veneer was thin. After taking the blood and sorting out the paperwork I returned to the office. The sergeant came in. "Well done doc. Now sit down, have a coffee and do not see anyone else until you've calmed down." He was right.

It did not feel like it at the time but I was lucky. If I had been practising in the early 60s there was no blood-alcohol limit. Doctors had to examine people and make an assessment; the old "walking a straight line" test.

By 1981 the technology had improved. As well as urine and blood, it was possible to measure alcohol in the breath accurately. It became an offence to have a level of alcohol in the breath greater than 35 mcg/100 mls. But the accurate breath testing machine, the Evidential Breath Testing device or "EBT, was at the police station. There was still a screening test at the roadside.

The EBT device was not introduced until 1983, as there needed to be extensive trials and extra training for the police. As with all drink-driving laws, the procedures had to be rock solid. There were plenty of drink-drivers who could afford expensive lawyers. Any weakness in the technology, and lawyers would find a way through.

Even then there was an extra safeguard called "the statutory option." Although the limit in the breath was set at 35 mcg, if it was between 35 mcg and 50 mcg the accused had a right to have a blood or urine test. It was up to the officer to decide whether the test should be blood or urine. With more accurate machines this "statutory option" has now been removed.

The new technology dramatically reduced my workload. Until 1983, I was called out to take blood from everyone accused of drink-driving. Suddenly, I was only called for borderline cases.

Any deviation from correct practice and the drink-driver would find the loophole. The officers had to follow a detailed proforma.

Mr Coates was a fifty-year-old, professional man who had been stopped by the police. He was driving erratically along the sea front. The suspicion was that he had been drinking.

At the station the Police officer asked various questions; had he used a mouth spray or had he eaten anything. He was then asked whether there is any medical reason why he "could not or should not provide a specimen of blood?" The officer was reading from the script.

Mr Coates claimed that he could not blow into the EBT device. This again was common. Sometimes drivers claim that they cannot blow, citing severe chest disease, such as asthma. I knew that asthma would have to be severe not to register breath on the machine but there can be long, difficult arguments in cases involving charges of failure to provide a specimen of breath. I did not have the medical records and so it was easier to accept his claim and take blood instead.

I saw him in the medical room with the officer in the case and explained my role and the limits of confidentiality. I could smell the drink and his eyes were red. The officer was inexperienced and unsure about the law but it did not matter. I was about to sit the Diploma of Medical Jurisprudence exam in London and had been hard at work revising. My homework had included becoming an expert on the law surrounding drinking and driving. The police also followed a standard protocol with the exact phrasing needed for each part of the case.

Mr Coates told me the name of his GP and told me that he also saw a psychiatrist who specialised in dealing with alcohol problems.

He was prescribed an antidepressant and "Antabuse"; a drug used to treat alcoholism. Antabuse reacts with alcohol so that anyone drinking would become ill, helping an alcoholic to stay dry. I did not want to prejudice the case by suggesting that it was not working.

He was not unusual. Many drink-drivers have an alcohol problem. They know that they will lose their licence if caught but they are never completely sober. They may even be unaware that drink has become a serious issue; it creeps up. A bottle of wine or a gin and tonic in the evening to "wind-down" becomes a habit. Gradually the drinking increases. They get angry if anyone suggests alcohol is becoming a problem but a conviction for drink-driving is an indicator that there may be a problem.

I was even rung by a GP colleague who told me that a friend of his had been caught drink- driving. He needed his licence. As an FME did I know a way around the system? I suggested the best way to really help his friend would be to accept that he could not drive for a while and get him help for his alcohol problem. I am not sure it was the answer he wanted.

Before I took the blood, Mr Coates claimed that he really could blow into the machine; the police had misunderstood. I let him have another go but the machine failed to register again.

I suggested that, as he was unable to blow, we take a blood sample. He said "I refuse" but held his arm out. Clearly this was not true consent and I explained that, if he refused to give a sample, he would be charged under section 7 of the Road Traffic Act 1988, for refusing to supply a sample. My revision was coming back to me. This, I explained, could have the same effect as a positive test. He would be fined and probably lose his licence. He still refused.

Two months later I received a phone call from the prosecuting solicitor. He asked me to explain the details again. After running through the story he pointed out that, although I was correct that refusal is an offence under Section 7, the law states that only a police officer can give this warning. The case was dropped. Luckily, I did pass the exam and used this as a case study.

He had got away with driving under the influence of alcohol although, as everyone is innocent until proven guilty, legally he was innocent. I still believe that no one is guilty unless they plead guilty or the evidence has been tested in court. This was not the end of the story. A few months later, I was called to the police station to take blood from a man who said he could not blow into the EBT device; it was Mr Coates, again. This time he agreed to have a blood sample taken and this time I got it right. Mr Coates did, eventually, lose his licence. His level proved to be more than two and a half times the legal limit. This meant that he had to join the "high risk offender scheme".

Since 1981 anyone who was over two and a half times the legal limit or refused to provide a specimen had to have a medical and blood tests before their licence could be returned. So if I had got it right the first time he would have been under the high risk offender scheme already, as he had refused to give a sample. In 1991 the scheme was extended to anyone who had two or more drink-drive convictions in ten years.

I knew that he would not get his licence back until he had further tests to exclude an alcohol problem. So, is he a criminal or a patient with the illness of alcohol dependence? By losing his licence he will get more help and the public will be protected.

I expect the high risk offender scheme applied to a drink-driver I was asked to see simply to assess whether he was fit to be detained.

He had already blown well over the 50 mcg needed for a conviction. The police had pulled him over after he had been driving erratically. When they opened the driver's door he fell out onto the road.

Another driver agreed to have blood taken but insisted that it was taken from his big toe. In other cases men have insisted the blood is taken from an even more intimate place. Although tempting to agree and reach for the largest needle, this would be unethical. If I had refused, could he have argued that he had not refused to give blood? Luckily the police were ready and pointed out a previous court ruling. If the doctor asks to take a blood sample "in accordance with general medical practice" and the accused refuses, that is still a refusal.

Luckily neither of these drivers had killed anyone. If they had they could be facing five years in prison. Before 1991 the crown prosecution service had a choice; either charge "death by dangerous driving", when alcohol was irrelevant, or charge with driving over the limit when the death would be irrelevant, although the presence of alcohol would affect the sentence. In 1992 a new law came into force of causing death by careless driving under the influence of drink or drugs. This now carries a statutory maximum punishment of fourteen years in prison.

I have heard a variety of excuses for refusing a sample, some better than others. One person claimed that he could not have a blood taken because he was a Jehovah's Witness. If he was a Jehovah's Witness he had not been listening. They refuse blood transfusions but do not have a problem with giving blood.

Another drunk-driver was covered in tattoos with earrings and studs in his nose and tongue – but claimed to have needle phobia.

This case was fairly clear-cut but, in most cases of needle phobia, we cannot know without notes or access to the GP. There are a few pointers. A discussion of foreign holidays can lead to an inadvertent admission of all the injections they needed. And, surprisingly, showing the needle to a true phobic leads to a fall in the pulse.

Judges have tried to clarify the situation. They ruled that, for a true needle phobia defence to run it has to mean that the person is physically or mentally unable to provide a sample without a risk to their health. "I don't like needles" is not enough. However, it can still be difficult.

In one case, the doctor did not accept that the driver had a valid excuse, as he simply claimed that blood tests made him feel faint. In court it turned out that he had a long history; including a panic attack when he cut himself shaving, fainting at the hairdresser's when a cut-throat razor was used and fainting at the GP's surgery when a blood test was even suggested. The problem for that particular doctor was that, with no notes, he had to make a judgement.

In the end I made a pragmatic decision. If any driver claimed to have a needle phobia I did not want to go to court and spend time arguing with a lawyer why his client could give blood, especially when I did not know his client and did not have any notes. It was easier and justice was more likely to be served, if I accepted the claim and took urine instead.

Drink-drivers cause accidents and are sometimes injured themselves and so I was often called to the hospital to take blood from defendants. In these cases I had to talk to the hospital doctor in charge first, and only if they agreed could I go ahead. Most A&E

doctors have seen the victims of drunk-drivers, and I was never refused unless there was a risk to the patient.

Occasionally, the alleged drunk -driver was still unconscious. This meant that it was not possible to get consent but, if we waited, the alcohol levels might have fallen. Luckily, the rules changed in 2002. I could then take blood for storage but it could not be analysed until the patient came round and gave consent.

Amazingly, some drunks claim that they have not been drinking. They, sometimes, claim that the alcohol was inhaled or spilt on their skin. In one case the defendant argued that he was over the limit because "someone spilt whisky on my cigarettes". The court did not accept that.

It may sound obvious but alcohol is taken as a drink by mouth. One drink-driver tried to argue that he had been decorating and had inhaled fumes which contained alcohol. It can be inhaled but research found that, despite several hours of inhaling an alcohol and air mixture in laboratory conditions, the maximum blood level achievable was only 50 mg. So it is not possible to go over the drink drive limit working with an alcohol spray. It is also not absorbed through the skin. Anyone over the drink-drive limit has drunk too much alcohol.

In several cases drivers have drunk alcohol after they were stopped, arguing that the high level of alcohol occurred after they were driving; the so-called "hip flask defence." As with any drug the level of alcohol in the blood goes up before it falls. By taking several readings over time and extrapolating back it is possible to see that the rise is inconsistent with drinking alcohol after they were stopped.

In one case the accused tried to argue that he had been inadvertently eating liqueur chocolates. Detailed research showed that it takes one kilogramme of liqueur chocolates to provide one unit of alcohol. An average man would need to eat about six to seven kilogrammes of liqueur chocolates to reach the limit. That would be difficult, even at Christmas.

In another case, the driver argued "my father was French." As the French are supposed to drink more than the British he claimed he could handle alcohol; wrong on almost every account. The French do not drink more than the British and the law simply specifies a level of alcohol above which it is illegal to drive. It does not matter whether you can "handle it."

One whispered to me, "They can't get me doc." I did not want to be pulled into a conspiracy but I let him continue.

"They can't take away my licence. I haven't got one" They did "get him." He was sent to prison.

Not every drink-driver was abusive or even alcoholic. Some simply misjudged the evening. They drove to meet friends and drank more than planned. "Go on – have one for the road."

I had some sympathy for the drivers who went out for an evening and arranged a taxi so that they did not drive home. They got to bed late, got up early and drove to work when still over the limit.

In one case I saw a driver who had just got back to the UK after a short-haul flight. At 30,000 feet it is easy to forget that you will be driving in an hour.

The situation is changing. The right of drink-drivers to opt for blood or urine if the breath test is between 40 mcg and 50 mcg has been removed so there will be even less work for the doctors or nurses. The machines are now accurate. Also the roadside machines may soon be effective enough to count as evidence without the need to check the level at the police station. Specially trained officers can now physically assess someone at the roadside.

So how can we reduce the road deaths from drink-drivers? Only Ireland, Malta and the USA have the same high limit of 80 mgs. Most countries, including Scotland, follow the advice of the European Union with a legal limit of 50 mg. In Estonia, Poland, Norway and Sweden it is 20 mgs and, in the Czech Republic, Hungary and Slovakia, the level is 0. Any alcohol in the blood when driving in Eastern Europe is illegal.

When the limit was cut in eight countries across Europe including Germany, France, Italy and Spain there was a ten point five per cent reduction in fatalities caused by drivers under fifty. By dropping the level from 50 mgs to 20 mgs Norway, Poland and Sweden cut fatal accidents by a further ten per cent. Stopping drivers at random also reduces accidents.

Drink-driving is dangerous for everyone but the road accident and fatality figures show that newly-qualified and young drivers are even more at risk. So should this be reflected in the law? Although both Ireland and the USA have the same high limit as the UK, they have low tolerance to drivers under 21, setting their limit at 10 mgs. Ireland also has a lower limit for new and commercial drivers.

The problem with having a different limit for young drivers is that it can send a message that it's OK to drive after some alcohol once you're over twenty one.

But no law will work if drink-drivers aren't caught. In the UK drivers are less likely to be stopped by the police than anywhere else in Europe. And this is reflected in public opinion. Some people believe they will get away with drinking and driving. Under the current law the police can stop drivers only if they believe they have committed a moving traffic offence. People are less likely to drink and drive if they know that, however carefully they drive, they might be stopped.

The Australians ran a poster campaign that read "If you drink and drive you're a bloody idiot". Change can come only through a cultural change in attitudes. The attitude to drinking and driving has changed since 1967. There may come a time when anyone caught drinking and driving, like Mr Coates, is seen to have an alcohol problem; an addiction or dependence when stopping alcohol would cause symptoms.

A man in his twenties was brought into the police station. He had been driving erratically but the breathalyser tested negative. The police told me that the car smelled of cannabis.

He was drowsy but relaxed. He had been clumsy and they were fairly sure that he had been driving under the influence of a drug, probably cannabis. But several hours had passed by the time he had been taken to the station, had been booked in and gone through the drink-drive procedure.

I had to find out whether he was driving whilst impaired through drink or drugs. This meant showing that he had taken a drug and that he was impaired; not always the same thing.

I used the standard proforma. I asked his medical and psychiatric history and whether he was prescribed any drugs.

I asked him to copy a paragraph from a book to test his handwriting. This is a useful test although one colleague was so tired in the night that he fell asleep and woke up to find the accused had written a whole page.

I ran through a neurological examination including the "Romberg test", asking him to stand and see how much he swayed when he closed his eyes, the "walk and turn" and the "finger-nose", touching my finger then his nose. I then gave an opinion.

Everything was normal. If he had taken cannabis the effects had worn off.

But the form simply asked the question *"is there a condition which might be due to a drug?"* From the examination the answer was no. Without any evidence from my examination that he had taken a drug I could not take a blood test. He was released.

Fortunately, this loophole has been closed. Now the question is whether there is a condition which *"at the time the detainee was alleged to have been driving might be due to a drug?"* As he was stopped by the Police because they believed that he had taken something the answer here would have been yes. So, unless the doctor finds a medical reason for their condition, a blood sample is taken. Even if the level of the drug is low it is possible to "back calculate" what the level would have been at the time of the offence.

I was called in one evening to see a heroin addict. She had injected, got in a car and driven into a roundabout. No one was hurt but she was clearly very drowsy.

She looked unkempt with old needle marks on her arms. There were no signs of drug withdrawal. But she knew where she was and I was confident that she understood the consent form, before signing it. I did not want her solicitor arguing that she did not consent to the examination so that all my evidence was inadmissible, as well as unethical.

I carried out the same examination and, this time, there was little doubt; she was "off her head". Despite terrible veins, I managed to get a sample and she was convicted.

Simply taking a drug does not make someone unfit, some people are more dangerous if they have not taken their medication. A severely depressed person is a safer driver if they have taken their anti-depressants and the depression is controlled. Equally the heroin addict might have been a safer driver and missed the roundabout if she had taken the prescribed dose of methadone rather than heroin. Withdrawal symptoms from heroin do not lead to safe driving; it is much saver to take the prescribed dose of methadone from a clinic.

The law has now changed so that the presence of an illegal drug when driving is an offence. Even for prescribed drugs the blood level must fit in with the prescribed dose.

Not all people brought in for driving impaired from a drug had taken anything at all.

I was called to the police station to see another man suspected of driving whilst unfit through drugs. "He's definitely on something, doc" the traffic officer explained but he had tested negative for alcohol.

He was talking continuously, although making very little sense. He could not sit still and seemed to believe that he had won the lottery. Clinically he was in the manic phase of bipolar disorder. I rang the duty psychiatrist. It turned out that he was well known to the psychiatric services. He did suffer from bipolar disorder and had stopped taking his medication. We arranged admission under the Mental Health Act.

The following week I received a phone call from the local authority. It turned out that he was a taxi driver. "Was he fit to return to work?" I had only seen him once when he was very unwell and could not answer. I suggested that they ask the psychiatrist or his own GP. I also wondered whether he had any passengers when manic. Far from being dangerous under the influence of drugs – his problem was that he was not taking his drugs.

In 1997, I naively hoped that attitudes might change following the death of Princess Diana. The evidence from the French Police and independent enquiry was clear. Her death was the result of getting into a car with a driver who had been drinking and who had then driven quickly through the streets of Paris. To make the situation even more perilous she had not worn a seat belt. Could some good come from the disaster? The public could see in graphic detail the results of drink-driving in the mangled wreck of the car. Sadly all that seemed to come out of it all were complicated and unnecessary conspiracy theories.

CHAPTER 7
JUST A SCRATCH

"Just a flesh wound"

– The Black Knight after his arms were cut off by King Arthur. Monty Python and the Holy Grail

In detective dramas the expert looks at an injury and, Sherlock Holmes's style, suggests it was inflicted by a knife from a right-handed man, of six feet two inches, from the left side at 23.00 hrs. In the real world, life was not so simple. For every expert who claimed that an injury had been inflicted in a certain way, there would be another expert who suggested something different.

Describing wounds forensically is not new. The Edwin Smith papyrus, written in ancient Egypt, in about 1600 BC, lists forty-eight cases involving wounds and trauma. Antistus, the ancient Roman "police surgeon", examined the body of the murdered Julius Caesar and proclaimed that only one of his twenty- three stab wounds caused his death. I'm not sure how this helped Caesar.

The first book on forensic medicine, Song Chi's *Collected Cases of Injustices Rectified or The Washing Away of Wrongs* was written in China in 1247. In it he says, "a forensic medical doctor must be serious, conscientious, and highly responsible", words which are equally important today.

Before seeing a certain Damien Caines, in custody, I was briefed by the Custody Sergeant. Damien had been brought in following a wounding. Allegedly, he had stabbed another man. This case could end up as Grievous Bodily Harm with intent or even attempted murder.

Bodily harm does not mean injury in the traditional sense. Harm includes anything which "*is calculated to interfere with the health or comfort of the victim*". Phrased in this way I wondered whether it should include some budget airlines.

And grievous means "really serious" harm. It was up to the lawyers to decide whether the injuries were "really serious", when he was indicted.

The issue of intent was also important for Damian. Inflicting GBH with intent carries a possible life sentence; whereas, inflicting unlawful wounding (without intent to inflict GBH) carries a sentence of up to five years in prison.

I saw Damien Caines at 08.50hrs in the medical room. He was my NHS patient and seemed relieved to see me. I explained that I was not seeing him as his GP but as an independent doctor. He was fully orientated but drowsy and aching. He denied taking any drugs or alcohol and was not suicidal. However, he smelled of drink.

At medical school I was not taught how to describe injuries forensically but I knew that the wrong terminology or failure to measure an abrasion properly could lead to confusion in court and undermine my credibility. I could hear a defence barrister saying "this doctor did not even know what a laceration is, ladies and gentlemen of the jury, so how can we rely on his other evidence beyond reasonable doubt?"

A good description relies on careful observation and a detailed understanding of the terminology. Previous generations of doctors were trained to examine patients in minute detail. They could not rely on an MRI scan or complicated blood tests. Today it is easy to slip into the habit of ordering tests, rather than spending time on detailed examinations. There is even a school of thought that clinical examinations are an out-dated waste of time.

Medical terminology is so confusing that even doctors can get it wrong. A study in the Netherlands showed, predictably, that forensic physicians were better than Emergency Room doctors, GPs and nurses at recognising injuries from photographs.

I took out a body chart and drew the four bruises on his chest, noting the size and position. I also drew the three-centimetre bruise on the back of his left hand and noted the multiple bruises on his left thigh. Unfortunately, I did not inherit my father's ability as a good amateur artist but I had a body map; outline drawings of parts of the body and others of the whole body, front and back.

Even describing a straightforward bruise was not easy. The simple definition is that it is an injury leading to damage under the skin; blood leaks out of the blood vessels and the skin turns blue. The problem with simple definitions is that they are usually wrong.

They are not always caused by damage. There can be "spontaneous bruises" in conditions such as haemophilia or with use of drugs such as warfarin or even aspirin. Some diseases such as meningococcal meningitis cause similar bleeding under the skin but these are not bruises but "purpura". It may sound impressive but the word is simply ancient Greek for purple.

We also know that some people, such as the elderly, bruise more easily. And different parts of the body bruise differently.

To make things even more confusing, there are different names for different size bruises. Bruises under five millimetres are called petechiae and larger ones ecchymoses.

Writing a statement or giving evidence in court the terms had to be correct. Defence barristers who specialised in the work knew the right terminology and were waiting to trip me up.

Bruises do not even have to occur at the site of injury. "Two lovely black eyes" are not always from trauma to the eyes. A hit on the top of the head can lead to blood travelling down the face and collecting around the eyes. If the bruising is around the actual eye and affects both eyelids it is unlikely the injury was to the eye. The eyeball itself is surrounded by bone. A fist to the eye will not penetrate into the eye but around it. A poke in the eye can damage the eyeball but it is unlikely to affect the lids.

Just to make life even more confusing, bruises are not instant.

I did not need an MRI scanner or tele-diagnosis, just a tape measure and magnifying glass; not the most sophisticated of equipment but vital for a competent examination. Each injury was accurately recorded, not only the size but also the position. Suggesting that a graze is five centimetres from the umbilicus or tummy button, would be useless. The umbilicus is mobile in people who are a little plump. . It needs to be measured from a fixed, bony point such as "five centimetres superior to the anterior, superior iliac spine" (the bone at the front of the pelvis). And I needed to remember that the police were also taking photos. In one case, an FME ended up in serious trouble because his markings on a body map did not match the police photos. The accused was found not guilty. How can anyone argue that the evidence is "beyond reasonable doubt" if the photographs and written descriptions do not match?

This was all before digital photography. Any photo taken by the police was taken twice, using two different cameras in case one of the films was damaged during processing. But today some doctors and nurses take their own photos with a digital camera or a smart phone. This opens up another discussion. Are the health care professionals' photographs a part of the prosecution evidence? Should they be released to the defence? Do they come under the Data Protection Act? There is no continuity of evidence, and so could they have been changed by editing software? I found it is easier to leave it to the experts.

There was a problem when a police surgeon took a series of forensic photos from an alleged assault and took the film to his local chemist to be developed. The chemist saw these explicit pictures and called the Police.

Physically my subject was well, with no sign of a serious head injury or drug withdrawal. I felt that it was safe to follow a "wait and see" policy, with the officers putting him on fifteen-minute observations.

I reviewed him again nine hours later at 17.00 hrs. This time he told me that he had been at home when he was hit with a bar stool before being beaten up. In the mêlée he stabbed someone. "It was about crack cocaine" he admitted. There was no alcohol involved.

He also admitted that he was taking diazepam 10 mgs three to four times a day and nitrazepam 5 mgs three to four at night. Both are benzodiazepine tranquilizers; both, highly addictive. I did not have access to his GP notes but, from memory, I did not think that these were prescribed drugs.

He also injected and smoked heroin, spending between £20 and £50 a day.

When I asked him how he felt he said "shitty." He was only out of prison three months. During the morning of the day before, he had seen his drugs' worker in the clinic and, in the afternoon, he had injected a £10 bag of heroin. At midnight he took two nitrazepam.

Checking him over again, he was still drowsy, with slurred speech. His pupils were a normal size and there was no other evidence of drug withdrawal.

I decided that he was fit to be detained. But were the injuries compatible with his version of events and his exercise of lawful self-defence?

Defensive injuries are usually on the palms of the hands and the forearms. A victim, on the ground, being kicked will often roll into a ball so that injuries are on the back, not usually the front of the chest and abdomen. Damien's injuries were not classic defensive injuries.

For Damien, my interpretation of the injuries could mean the difference between a conviction of GBH with intent and a long sentence of imprisonment, or acquittal on the grounds of self-defence. However, interpreting injuries is difficult and, potentially, dangerous. Just describing an injury is not always helpful to a court. Judges and juries could say "so what?" The court expects the doctor to explain "what" (bruise, laceration etc.), "where" (a detailed description of where the injury is, preferably with a body map), "when" (a rough idea of the age of the injury) and, finally, "how." It is the "how" which causes most difficulty and could land the doctor in trouble. Interpretation can be subjective.

These were not typical defensive injuries but detailed interpretation was difficult. In the end, I was not called to court. My evidence was not contested and probably not important. The witnesses and history were vital. He was found guilty of GBH with intent and sent to prison for seven years. Was the court biased against a heroin addict or was this verdict reasonable? I was not in court to hear the arguments.

Terminology can be confusing. Even the word "injury" does not have a clear meaning. If it is a physical problem, where does that leave the whole industry of personal injury lawyers? Legally, injury could include "*any disease and any impairment of (the) physical or mental condition*. "But if I shouted "*come quickly, he's seriously injured*" no one would expect to find a patient with a deteriorating mental condition.

"Wound" does have a legal definition, although it is does not always match the meaning used in everyday language. As far back as 1834 it was ruled that it is only a wound if the skin is broken. So, if the skin is intact, as in a bruise, it is not a wound. If I had used the word "wound" to describe Damien's bruises the defence barrister would have been keen to point out my incompetence.

A Police Surgeon's Lot

In a historical case, the victim was hit just above the eye by a pellet from a gun. There was severe internal bleeding but, as the pellet had not actually penetrated both layers of the skin, the court ruled that this was not a wound. To the general public this must seem bizarre. "He's been shot, with massive internal bleeding, but was not wounded".

Ageing of bruises is also a challenge. In one case, an alleged assault took place on a Friday night and I saw the victim on the following Sunday. In court, the defence barrister tried to pin me down.

"Were these bruises inflicted on the Friday or could it have been earlier or later?"

I explained the problem and how difficult it is to age bruises.

If there is yellowing around the bruise, it is probably over sixteen hours old; beyond that it is impossible. Even the textbooks give different accounts of the colour bruises go through at different stages.

In one study of childhood bruising, a hospital doctor, a staff nurse and a photographer examined fifty-eight bruises. There was complete agreement on the colour in only twenty seven per cent of cases examined and in twenty four per cent of photographs. In two-thirds of cases the descriptions did not match the photograph. Descriptions of bruises are not consistent.

In another study, experts were asked to look at photographs of bruises produced by a suction pump on the upper arms on eleven volunteers. The results, again, showed that dating bruises is, at best, unreliable, especially if the bruise is over twelve hours' old. Even some "experts" were completely wrong. Things improved slightly when they were asked to assess bruises on the same person, in chronological order.

Accordingly, when I was pressed, I sat on the fence. This story became headline news in my local paper and I was quoted, *"The doctor said that the bruises were either inflicted at the time or before, or after."* I'm not sure whether that helped the court but it was accurate.

I always avoided expressions such as "fingertip bruising" as it implies a cause but it is used by some colleagues simply to describe small circular bruises. I was once pressurised to interpret bruises described by a colleague as fingertip bruises. I am not usually quick-witted in court. There is too much pressure. However, this time, I managed a reply that appeared to stump the barrister.

"Surely, doctor, these bruises must be caused by fingertips. Why else would they be called fingertip bruises?"

"Not necessarily". I replied, "After all, tennis elbow is not usually caused by tennis. It's just a name."

Occasionally the injuries were simply not compatible with the story. Robbie was well known to the police for joy riding. He had a habit of stealing cars. The police found a car smashed into a wall. There was no driver but Robbie was seen running away. When he was caught, I was asked to see him. He had a linear forty centimetre tender area across his chest with a few abrasions. At least he had the sense to put on a seat belt when he drove stolen cars but he denied stealing or driving the crashed car.

"So", I asked, "how did you get the chest injury?"

"It's me girl friend" he explained. "She gave me a French kiss right across my chest." I would like to have seen this girl with forty centimetre wide lips.

During the interview, he admitted the obvious; he had stolen the car and crashed it.

One of the problems with seeing him so soon after the accident was that the bruises had not yet appeared. Occasionally I would arrange to see the person again and find new bruises appearing.

A century earlier, the delay in the appearance of bruises nearly sent a young woman to the scaffold. In 1894 Marie Hermann, a prostitute, was accused of murdering Henry Stevens. She argued that it was self-defence; he was trying to strangle her and she grabbed a nearby poker and hit him. Initially, there was no evidence of any marks on her neck. The case against her was strong, especially in the days of all male juries. Very few men had sympathy for prostitutes in Victorian London. But her barrister, Sir Edward Marshall Hall QC ('The Great Defender'), went to see the matron of Holloway Prison, where she was remanded. Bruises had now appeared on her neck, which fitted the story of a man's hand gripping her neck tightly. As well as defending her profession by pointing out that "these women are what men made them" he arranged for the Holloway matron to give evidence. The case is also famous for his plea to the jury: "Look at her, gentlemen – God never gave her a chance – won't you?"After only 45 minutes, the jury acquitted her of murder and saved her from the gallows.

In one of my cases a woman alleged that her knickers had been forced down before she was raped. There was evidence of recent intercourse and fingernail type scratches on her thighs. It appeared to be a serious and unpleasant case.

Forensically a graze is called an abrasion but even this is not straightforward. If it is long with little width it becomes a scratch.

By looking at the scratch carefully with my magnifying glass it was possible to see that the skin was rolled up at one end. This gave an idea which direction the scratch was inflicted. It was upwards. When this was put to her she admitted that she had had consensual intercourse, then a row with her partner. She had scratched her own legs, before calling the police.

In another case, a doctor working in the Accident and Emergency department was torn apart in the witness box over the word "laceration." He explained, wrongly, that it is the medical term for any type of cut. All the lawyers in the court knew the definition; the only professional who did not know was the doctor.

Lacerandum is Latin for 'tear'; nothing to do with a cut. A laceration is a full thickness tear to the skin caused by a blunt instrument. A knife would only cause a laceration if the handle hit the victim. Again the magnifying glass comes in useful. The wound is rarely straight; the edges are jagged with some bruising. There may be tissue crossing the wound.

Many doctors who should know better get this wrong, including some A&E consultants. There was even a picture on the front of the prestigious British Medical Journal wrongly labelled a laceration. This led to a flood of letters from pedantic forensic doctors.

A cut is exactly what is says on the tin, a cut. Looking closely, picking up the magnifying glass, it is possible to look at the edges to decide whether the knife had straight edges or was serrated. We can also work out the direction of the cut. Usually the first cut is the deepest (to coin a phrase) with the cut getting less deep as the knife was removed.

A stab wound is a cut that is deeper than its length. Sometimes the television detective puts the knife by the stab wound and declares that the wound is too small to have been inflicted by that knife. He has forgotten that skin is elastic. When a knife is withdrawn the hole can shrink leaving a wound, which appears smaller than the knife.

Luckily gunshot wounds are rare in the UK. In 2012 there were over four hundred killings by police using firearms in the USA and none in the UK. The USA had eleven thousand and seventy-eight homicides from firearms in 2010 compared with fifty- one in the UK in 2012. So America has eighty- three gun deaths a day, the UK has fifty- one a year.

When Roy Jenkins was the British home secretary he was asked by an American, "Why don't you arm your police?" He answered, "Why do you arm your criminals?"

The only serious injury I have seen from a firearm was in an A&E department, when I was a junior doctor. A man had been out shooting on Dartmoor and came home to find his wife in bed with another man. He shot the man dead and then turned the gun on himself, putting the barrel in his mouth and firing. It took out his cheek and eye but missed his brain.

As he was wheeled in with a drip up and a pad over what was left of his face the paramedic turned to me and said, "He's tried an overdose before but this looks like more than a cry for help."

After surgery from the neurosurgeons, orthopaedic surgeons and plastic surgeons, his only lasting injury was the loss of one eye. As a junior doctor, I was not involved in any forensic assessment, although I did hear that he recovered, was transferred to prison and eventually found guilty of murder.

Having discussed injuries, what about the significance of an absence of injuries? Can that be significant?

I saw an alleged murderer in the custody centre. There had been a party that a man gate-crashed. He was beaten up and, when on the ground, the defendant allegedly kicked him in the head; causing an injury which proved fatal. The defence admitted that he had killed the man but suggested that it was a 'tragic accident'; there had been a fight but it was manslaughter, not murder. Murder carries an automatic life sentence.

I had examined him, head to toe, and could not find the slightest mark. In court, the defence team found it difficult to find any convincing arguments that he had been in a fight, in which the other man was killed, but he had escaped without a single mark on his body. However, the prosecution case, that wearing large boots and kicking someone in the head does not injure the assailant, was strong. He was found guilty of murder. Lack of injury was crucial.

Nicola was a patient in my GP practice. She was typical of many women in the area; in her mid-thirties living in a typical three bedroom semi-detached house. Her three children attended the local primary school and she only came to the surgery occasionally for routine cervical smears and family planning. Her husband worked as a middle manager in a local building firm.

She came to see me with a series of vague symptoms: tiredness, poor sleep and lower abdominal pain. I examined her and ran a series of blood tests, all of which were normal.

The follow up appointment was on a hot August day but I noticed that she was wearing a roll neck jumper and long sleeves. She also failed to make eye contact. Perhaps alarm bells should have rung but I decided simply to review her in a week's time. I remember my GP trainer telling me "you don't have ten minutes with the patient, you have twenty years."

The following week she was more withdrawn and thought that she was wasting my time. I asked to check her blood pressure, not because I needed to know; she had her blood pressure taken every time she came for the contraceptive pill. It gave me a chance to look at her arms.

At the top of her arms was a series of small bruises, typical of a grip, with the mark from a thumb on the inside and four marks from fingers on the outside.

"How did you get these" I asked.

"I must have knocked myself gardening." The story did not match the injury.

I then asked to see her neck. She reluctantly pulled down the roll neck to show more bruises. Some were yellowing, some appeared fresh. She was the victim of violence and the most likely cause was domestic violence, sometimes called "intimate partner violence." I knew that the other classical injuries would be to her breasts and abdomen but felt that it would be too intrusive to suggest such a thorough examination. One computer programme designed to help doctors pick up cases lists two hundred and fifty symptoms. Some may not be obvious.

There are numerous statistics thrown around, including by the World Health Organization, suggesting that one third of women globally are victims. The figures can be challenged in academic circles but, for a woman who is terrified and facing serious injury or even death, it would not matter if she were the only case in the world. She needed help and support. At least she had come to see me. Abused women might not wish to go to the surgery or A&E with obvious injuries.

I was fairly sure that I was dealing with a case of domestic violence but, if I challenged her, she might not return or she might come back with her husband, making it impossible to ask questions. Often powerful abusers join their partner in the A&E department or GP's surgery and take over the consultation, not allowing the victim to speak. They can be charming and appear caring to win over the professional.

To add to the difficulty, she may be terrified. How will her husband react if he finds out that she has been talking about him? He may have told her that no one would believe her. He is far more credible. Sadly, that is often true. She may even believe him when he tells her that she "deserved it". He probably apologised and told her that it will not happen again. She wanted to believe him.

I arranged to see her again. I could have been wrong or the abuse could be from someone else; not her husband. But, if I had missed it, she would be at serious risk of injury or even death as well as a four to five-fold increased risk of mental health problems, especially anxiety, depression, alcohol and drug abuse or post traumatic stress disorder.

I had a word with the Health Visitor. She could run some background checks; had anyone else expressed concern? How were the children doing at school?

The following week Nicola was openly upset. The Health Visitor had been round and helped her open up. I just allowed her to talk.

"He doesn't mean to" she started. I did not break the silence. "He's a good man really. Perhaps I deserved it."

I made it clear that I believed her and that she was not alone. She was brave to bring it up.

"It is clearly not your fault." I let the words hang in the air. "You don't have to put up with this, you know". It was the beginning. I saw her regularly and also gave her the number for a local group who support victims of domestic violence. Eventually, she gained enough confidence and support to leave him but still did not want to tell the police. She still loved him, just hated what he did. Her emotional injuries were worse than the physical ones.

I also learnt that domestic violence is not new. In 1891, at the age of 24, Emmeline Pethick-Lawrence travelled to London to work as a volunteer at the West London Methodist Mission. In her biography, written in 1938, "My Part in a Changing World" she described how she wrote: *"Drunkenness was extremely common... It seemed for many the only refuge from depression and misery. The effect of drunkenness upon the ordinary relationship of husband and wife, parents and children, was disastrous"*

Domestic violence, fuelled by alcohol, was common and accepted. *"There was a particular point of view with regard to wife-beating. A friend of mine was once walking along the street and she passed a woman with a black eye. At the same time two other women passed, and one of them remarked: "Well, all I can say is, she is a lucky woman to have a husband to take that trouble with her." Another woman who had gone through a similar experience remarked: "Well, it ain't pleasant to be knocked about, but the making-up is lovely."*

Looking at the "Andy Capp" cartoons from the 1960s, Andy Capp's wife, Flo, is often seen with bruises and stars around her head as a part of the "joke."

And injuries to children can create even more problems. Whenever there is a tragedy the popular press make the diagnosis of child abuse sound easy. It is easy in hindsight. Every report into every tragedy comes to the same conclusion. The key to picking up abuse and saving children is communication.

I had a niggling concern about Kyle. She was eighteen months old but, somehow, did not always react like a toddler. There was nothing specific. All her milestones were normal and she lived with both her parents. Dad was a fairly dominant character who usually came in with Kyle and her Mum and he did most of the talking.

At nine months' old she had a strange mark on her head. X-ray showed an abnormality on the skull and the films were sent away to an expert at a large teaching hospital. There was no clear answer except that it was not a serious problem.

One morning I received a phone call from the GP who had been on duty overnight. He had been called out to see Kyle for a minor viral illness but came away worried. Normally overnight visits were faxed through but he asked to talk to me.

"I wanted to talk to you about this one," he explained. "There was nothing to find and the child was not ill but I've got a gut feeling that there's something else going on." Here was an experienced GP with no evidence but enough "gut feeling" to talk to me personally.

I contacted the health visitor and we had a meeting later in the day. We went through all the records. Kyle had numerous consultations, all for minor problems. It was not clear why her mother kept bringing her. All first time Mums worry and I saw it as a part of my role as a GP to help them through the normal anxieties of parenthood, but this case seemed different.

I spoke to the paediatrician and arranged for Kyle to go to the hospital for a full skeletal survey; x-raying the whole body. Her mother agreed. I wondered whether she was also relieved.

X-rays showed seventeen fractures of different ages. Kyle was admitted to hospital and both parents were arrested. Both denied causing any injury and both blamed the other parent. Social services found out that the father had moved down from another part of the country after a child from a previous relationship had been found to have multiple injuries. It had not been clear how those injuries had been caused and no one was charged.

For Kyle there was not enough evidence to prove either parent was the abuser beyond reasonable doubt. They were both released with no charge. Kyle was eventually adopted. I do not know what happened to her parents but I hope that the father has not settled elsewhere with a new partner and new baby.

CHAPTER 8
THE DRUG SCENE

We can no more hope to end drug abuse by eliminating heroin and cocaine than we could alter the suicide rate by outlawing high buildings or the sale of rope"

Ben Whittaker (The global fix)

In the 1970s I knew very little about the illegal drug scene. Admitting a heroin addict to hospital I asked "do you ever use barbiturates?"

"No, I reckon they are dangerous." He was right, they are dangerous but injecting heroin was also not a safe option. This was my introduction to the problems of street drugs.

Even when I started as a police surgeon I had to look up the withdrawal symptoms of heroin; knowledge which became fundamental to my work only ten years later.

By the 1980s and 1990s it was not possible to work as an FME without some understanding of the drug scene. Torquay may have appeared as a quaint, Victorian, seaside resort but, under the surface, we faced a major drug problem. For most youngsters this was just a phase they passed through and very few came to any harm but about one in ten became "a problem drug user" injecting or dependant.

There was a subculture of drug use across society. One group were the clubbers or cannabis smokers who bought their drugs with their own legitimate money. Their only crime was possession of an illegal drug.

At the heavy end, addicts used heroin, amphetamines or prescribed drugs blagged off doctors. Cocaine was less common in South Devon in the 1980s and 1990s as it was too expensive. I only came across it a few times when more wealthy holidaymakers came down. It was being used by the 1980s' city bankers, the "Yuppies", not the homeless burglars in Devon.

Back in 1971, before I started as a police surgeon, drugs which could be abused were classified into A, B or C, depending on how dangerous they were to the individual and to society as a whole. These were called "controlled drugs."

Politicians found regulating recreational drugs difficult. They were not experts and any move to allow a drug, whatever the evidence, was met with "soft on drugs" by the popular press so they set up the Advisory Committee on the Safety of Drugs. The final classification into class A, B or C drugs was not made by politicians but based on advice from the committee made up from experts in the field.

The classification of different drugs from A to C was irrelevant to my work as a GP. I still carried diamorphine or heroin in a fishing box in the back of my car. It was a useful pain killer but, as a police surgeon, I was aware of the dangers if this drug should ever reach the streets. In 1985 the Misuse of Drugs regulations were introduced which tightened up the rules on who could carry and prescribe controlled drugs, and an unlocked fishing box definitely did not figure. Prescriptions had to be hand written in both words and figures to reduce the risk of fraud. This separated drugs into schedules one to five. This had no bearing on whether they are more or less dangerous than other controlled drugs.

Schedule one were the drugs with no medical use such as cannabis and LSD. Even as a doctor I could only possess these if undertaking research and with a licence from the Home Office.

As the problem with street drugs increased I had to be more careful in my daily surgery. Prescription pads could be stolen and people would come to the surgery to try to "blag" drugs.

Often they would claim terrible pain and ask for strong morphine or codeine painkillers. In one case I prescribed an anti inflammatory tablet, which would have been effective for genuine pain. He ripped up the prescription and threw it at me. I took this as a subtle hint that this was not the medication he was after.

Another one threatened violence in the waiting room. The only solution was to call the police. They arrived, arrested him and he was taken to the custody centre. Within half an hour I had a call from the custody sergeant.

"We've got an addict here, doc, who's asking to see you. He says he's withdrawing and needs medication."

I arrived to find the same person who had been arrested in my surgery. After checking him over and finding no evidence of drug withdrawal I explained "you're still not getting anything."

The drugs were not always the obvious ones. I had several addicts claiming that they were about to cross to Ireland or France and needed something to stop seasickness. They had worked out that some anti-sickness medication enhanced the effects of heroin.

One of my colleagues was told that some sleeping tablets he had prescribed had ended up on the streets. He was an excellent, caring GP. He was not naive and knew the risks so how had he been conned?

At the end of each consultation an elderly lady who visited his surgery regularly would ask, "Oh Doctor. Please could I have a few more of those wonderful sleeping tablets? You're so kind."

The police investigation found that she was then selling them on via her grandson to supplement her pension. As my colleague said if a young man covered in tattoos asks for "sleepers" he would be careful but it never occurred to him that he was being conned by a little old lady.

The only time we had problems with one of our prescriptions was when I received a phone call from a chemist. A drug addict had torn off a blank prescription from a printer in another surgery and stolen a surgery stamp from us. This stamp was not used on prescriptions but on forms and private sick notes. It was clearly the wrong stamp. And each prescription on a printer has a code number so that it could be traced. The addict had written "Diazepam 10 mgs 100" on the prescription and, where the script was "signed" he wrote my partner's name. Another "give away" was that it was legible. It was not the most sophisticated of forgeries and he was soon arrested but it did make us tighten up security. I stopped leaving the surgery stamps around and we put security locks on the doors so that no one could walk into a consulting room and steal prescriptions from the printers. The actual prescription pads were always kept under lock and key.

But most illegal drugs in the Bay were not blagged from GPs.

"The grandmother heroin dealer" was how the local paper described her. She had also been my GP patient for years. When I visited her I found her terraced house had large security locks on all the doors and bars on the windows, despite being in the middle of Torquay. She was always friendly and co-operative but the excessive security fitted in with the rumours I had heard regarding her "business."

The house was impregnable to both addicts and the Police. In the door was a small slot. The police suspected that a large amount of the heroin used on the streets came from her. They watched people knocking on her door, handing over cash and walking away with wraps of heroin. The secret surveillance had probably recorded my visits although, hopefully, they did not think I was involved.

The police could have arrested the users but this would not have stopped the supply. They suspected her supply was coming down the motorway from Liverpool. She was the "middleman" working with some major dealers.

She was arrested several times but the Police could not make the allegations stick. She even featured in the local paper as a victim of police harassment as well as complaining to me about the terrible police. I was not sure whether she knew about my other work.

Whenever there was a raid, by the time the police had managed to get in, there were no drugs to be found.

One day she came to see me quite upset. Her son had been sent to prison "just because he had a bit of cannabis." This seemed excessive until I read the report in my local paper. He did have "a bit of cannabis" but also a substantial amount of cash and some weighing scales. The evidence that he was dealing was impressive. Maybe he was following in the family tradition.

Finally the police were successful. The intelligence suggested that she had buried the drugs in her garden. As they dug they first found some cannabis. Her plan was that she would be arrested for cannabis dealing and that they would not keep digging to find the heroin underneath.

But even for cannabis, a class B drug, possession with intent to supply can lead to 14 years in prison. Intent to supply does not necessarily mean a dealer. Having a bit of weed to give to your mates is possession with intent to supply, even if no money changes hands.

The police kept digging. Eventually they found the heroin. Possession with intent to supply a Class A drug and can lead to life imprisonment and an unlimited fine. She was sent to prison for eight years. Even simple possession of a Class A drug can lead to 7 years in prison.

I saw her again after she was released on parole but then the prison contacted the local police. They had found evidence of her dealing drugs in prison. She was to be recalled immediately. The

Police explained that they could not arrest her now because she was back in another prison. After release she had reopened for business but, this time, the police managed to convince the court quickly.

The addicts buying heroin from this grandmother had no idea what they were buying. Dealers cut the powder to increase supply and make more money. In the 1990s the police started testing for drugs on some people arrested for other offences. This would not mean further charges for drug-related offences. Although possession of a controlled drug is an offence, it is not an offence to have the drug in your blood.

One of the surprises was to see angry drug addicts who had tested negative. They had just spent £10 on a wrap of heroin, injected it, been arrested and were negative – the wrap obviously contained no heroin.

However, it was one of the worst aspects of the job seeing so many deaths from accidental overdoses. Drugs bought on the street do not have the British standard kite mark and, if the exact strength is not certain, addicts end up taking a dose that is too strong.

This uncertainly made the drug scene even more dangerous. If I have a headache I might take paracetamol. I know that paracetamol bought in the UK is safe if it is taken responsibly. There is quality control from the manufacture of the chemicals through to the tablets and packaging. I know that 500 mgs of paracetamol will be 500 mgs of paracetamol. And the inactive bulk of the tablet will be inactive and safe. I can even look up the manufacturer and, if there is a problem, the product can be traced.

If I were offered a paracetamol tablet that had been manufactured illegally, no idea where it was made, no idea whether it really contained 500 mgs of paracetamol and no idea what else I might be swallowing I would not take it. I would rather put up with my headache; not because paracetamol is dangerous but because this tablet carries an unknown and unacceptable risk.

The same problem applied to all street drugs, not just heroin. There were debates whether, for example, ecstasy really is more dangerous than legal drugs such as alcohol. However, a punter buying an ecstasy tablet on the streets or in the clubs might not be buying ecstasy; the dose might be inconsistent in different tablets, or it might contain other, dangerous chemicals.

The CID were excited. Torquay was about to hit the headlines with the largest ecstasy seizure in the country. They knew the main dealer and followed him to his supplier in The Netherlands. He was allowed through customs in a sting operation. They waited until he had arrived back in Torquay before they raided his flat and found a large number of tablets, ready for sale around the clubs. The raid was made easier as his flat was opposite the police station.

The tablets looked real but, when analysed, they only contained saccharine. He had been conned by his Dutch dealer. Smuggling saccharine into the country is not an offence and he was released. He must have had mixed feelings but, if he had not been caught, at least he would not have caused any harm selling saccharine in the clubs. I suspect that the clubbers would have found the "ecstasy" highly effective from the placebo effect.

Adulterated drugs can cause real harm. One Sunday morning, a man was brought in to the station, under section 136 of the Mental Health Act. He had been behaving strangely, standing on the sea front waving down cars. He believed that every car was full of policemen and, eventually, he was right. But then we had another person brought in, also suffering hallucinations, with bizarre thoughts.

It turned out that, the night before, a dealer had been selling "ecstasy" tablets in a club that were not ecstasy but dihydrocodeine with drops of LSD impregnated. These would probably have cost the dealer more than ecstasy and it is a mystery why he should choose to give clubbers a trip but it explained the apparent epidemic of bizarre mental illness on a Sunday morning.

As I was treating more people with drug problems so I needed to understand the general principle behind all addiction; whether it is to drugs, gambling or anything else. Many of these people wanted an instant result. With drugs or gambling the quicker the "hit" and the quicker it wears off, the more addictive the activity. Betting on the National Lottery and waiting until the draw on Wednesday or Saturday is less addictive than Internet or slot machine gambling when the results are instant. Crack cocaine, which acts almost immediately but can wear off in twenty minutes, is more addictive than cocaine powder.

The first aim in treatment was to help the addict move from a quick acting drug to one that lasts far longer. Heroin addicts were treated with methadone, a drug that lasts over 24 hours. Many people in the police cells were taking drugs prescribed by their GP. Ideally I asked the prisoner whether I could ring the GP but not everyone was detained during office hours.

Some of these prisoners had traditional medical problems such as heart disease or diabetes. Even here the staff could not just give the medication. I would need to check and discuss it with the patient. And I had to leave clear, written instructions for the staff. Prisoners might even refuse their medication in the hope that they would end up in hospital. One diabetic burglar always refused his insulin in the hope that I would send him to hospital. I never did. I knew he would soon be in court and then either get home for his insulin or get it in prison. But he tried the same trick every time he was arrested. He never learned.

Things could go wrong, even with clear, written instructions. On one occasion, I saw a drug addict who was withdrawing and so I gave him some medication. I then wrote him up for more medication later on. Unfortunately I did not make it clear that I had given the tablets and the staff gave him more drugs immediately I left. He did not come to any harm; as an addict he was probably delighted. He certainly did not tell the staff that he had already had his drugs. It was, however, my fault; I had not made it clear.

Any treatment programme, whether for heart disease, diabetes or drug addiction, needed to be continued. However, when people brought in their own medication we could never be sure whether it was prescribed, stolen or bought on the streets.

Therefore, anyone with any medication needed to be seen by a doctor or nurse. We needed to look at it carefully; was it clearly labelled with the patient's name? Was it dated? Sometimes addicts blagged a small number of pills from a GP and filled the bottle or packet with drugs bought on the streets. I have seen a full bottle of tablets that were clearly labelled for ten tablets with a date six months earlier and the detainee's name. Occasionally the tablets were even different colours.

One of my colleagues was shown a bottle of antibiotic capsules with the correct name. The amoxicillin capsules were genuine; yellow and red with powder inside. The detainee was given his medication regularly until it was discovered that, before arrest, he had emptied all the antibiotic powder from the capsules and replaced it with cocaine. He was inadvertently being given cocaine three times a day by the custody staff.

It is unethical for any professional to argue "I don't prescribe for druggies". All the detainees were our patients who had a right to be treated appropriately for any medical problems, whether it was heart disease, diabetes or drug addiction. But we did have a "six hour rule." We did not give any drugs used for addiction such as tranquillizers or opiates until the detainee had been in custody for at least six hours. This is not to "make them suffer" but we did not know whether they had taken anything before arrest. There was a real danger that, by prescribing too soon, we could inadvertently be giving an overdose. But even the "six-hour rule" was not cast in stone. To give or withhold medication was always a clinical decision based on a careful history and examination.

I had to be careful. One detainee had only been with us a short time and so was refused medication. Unfortunately, I had not been told that he had been transferred from another police station and had actually been in custody for twenty-four hours.

Callum was arrested driving erratically. On booking in he denied having taken any drugs. After booking in he blew negative for alcohol and was assessed by the FME for drugs. Blood was taken which later proved negative.

After three hours, he suddenly collapsed. Despite cardiopulmonary resuscitation or CPR from paramedics, the FME and the police, he died in custody.

Post mortem examination found numerous ecstasy tablets wrapped in cling film. The blood levels of ecstasy at death were incompatible with life. But the blood in the earlier sample only showed a small trace of ecstasy.

There were no tests that could have completely excluded "stuffed" drugs. In a French study of fifty body-stuffers, the drug was only detected in the urine in fifty-seven per cent of the detainees. Plain X-ray only showed thirty-three per cent of swallowed wraps. . A simpler way of assessing whether drugs might be in the gut is by giving the detainee sweet corn. When it appeared in the stool we knew that anything in the gut had passed through.

The IPPC (Independent Police Complaints Commission) investigated. He was recorded on the booking-in video denying having taken any drugs but the IPPC still asked questions. Did he have some powder around his mouth? Should the police have realised the risk? Luckily I was not the FME involved. He received a thank you letter from Callum's family, who understood that he had done everything possible but the IPPC were not so supportive. After a grilling he was completely exonerated. The letter clearing him of any responsibility for the death ended with the reassuring words: "we have decided not to take criminal action against you." He had no idea that criminal action was being considered. He nearly gave up forensic work.

Technically Callum was a "body-stuffer," swallowing unwrapped or poorly wrapped drugs rapidly to avoid detection immediately before arrest.

Occasionally I saw body-pushers. These people were often dealers who inserted drugs into the rectum or vagina wrapped more carefully, so that they could carry the drugs around without being detected.

After our experience with Callum, if anyone was suspected of stuffing drugs we did not want them in custody; they should be observed in hospital. But there was a problem. A&E departments discharged them once they had been assessed. The fact that they were sitting on a time bomb did not merit admission. If the patient dropped dead, as happened to Callum, the A&E department did not appear worried. I tried to point out that, if a patient had a large aortic aneurysm, at risk of bursting, they would not discharge him, even if all the observations were normal – but it fell on deaf ears.

Even if the hospital did keep the patient, what would happen if they refused to stay? The hospital had no legal power to keep the patient but taking them back to custody was not safe.

Intelligence from other forces found that our policy was causing problems. Dealers knew that, if they stuffed drugs, they would not be kept in custody and could walk out of hospital. What better way to smuggle drugs into Devon and Cornwall?

Throughout medicine, we balance risk against benefit. Here we had the same problem. If drugs could be brought in freely, there was a serious risk to our local population but, if we detained the dealers in custody, we might have another death.

Luckily, research came to our aid. In a review of 180 papers between 1950 and 2006, in which 21 were considered relevant, it was reported that, "Body stuffers or packers who have no risk factors for complications and are asymptomatic at six hours post-ingestion may be safely discharged from hospital with instructions to seek further medical advice." So it was safe to have them in custody after six hours. If a disaster occurred, we had good evidence to support our decision.

Working in a provincial custody centre I did not see any "body-packers." These are more likely to be found at airports, packing drugs in condoms, latex or rubber packets and transporting them across international boundaries.

In the 1980s, a female patient of mine was arrested, suspected of packing drugs in her vagina. We had to follow both the law and medical ethics. And they were not always the same. Legally a doctor could examine a detainee accused of stuffing or packing drugs but only under strict rules; known as an "intimate search". This search could only be carried out if looking for class A drugs "with intent to supply" or for weapons.

The examination had to be authorised by a senior police officer and take place in medical premises. If a package should burst we needed a full resuscitation team.

The detainee had to agree. Even this was contentious. In the 1980s the Home Office advised that a doctor could examine someone against their will if the police suspected that they had packed drugs but the General Medical Council ruled that any intimate examination, without consent, would be gross professional misconduct. So, legally, it was possible but I would then be stuck off. Not a great choice.

Everything was set up. I saw her in the cell but her solicitor had agreed for us to go ahead with an intimate search; the hospital agreed that we could carry this out in the A&E department and it was authorised by a superintendent. I just had to explain everything to the patient.

"I understand that you've agreed to this." I said, after running through the plans.

"Yes" she said, "the police say it is the only way that I am going to get out of here." I knew I would not be popular but this was not freely given consent. In court it would be argued, correctly, that it was under duress. I could not go ahead. I spoke to her solicitor and the procedure was cancelled.

The law is now clearer. Legally, as well as ethically, a search cannot be carried out without consent but, now, the court can "draw an inference" if a defendant refuses. When the law was changed I wondered whether telling someone that, if they refuse, the court could "draw an inference" was also consent under duress.

The UK spends £1.2 bn a year on drug law enforcement and treatments. If we include the cost to the police, courts and prisons, it probably exceeds £4 bn. However, the cost to the economy could be greater. Addicts steal to feed their habit. These are costs we all pay, through increased house insurance and prices on the high street. It is impossible to get firm figures but it has been estimated that the total cost of the illegal drug problems to the UK economy is around £16 bn a year. Illegal drugs are expensive. There was one drug which caused more problems than any other – alcohol. And I will discuss this in the next chapter.

CHAPTER 9
PROBLEMS WITH BOOZE

"Alcohol leads to nose painting, sleep and urine. Lechery, sir it provokes and unprovokes ... it provokes the desire but it takes away the performance."

Shakespeare, Macbeth

On 8th October 2002, a man was brought into the enquiry office of Torquay Police Station by a member of the public concerned for his welfare. He did not manage to answer any of the questions from the officer at the desk and was clearly at risk. It would have been dangerous to send him back on to the streets and so he was arrested for drunkenness. In hindsight he should have been sent to hospital, although he may have been discharged as "just a drunk".

He was carried into the custody suite. The custody sergeant took him straight into a video cell. I was already in the police station and was asked to see him immediately.

He was overweight, grunting and unconscious. As I was checking his "observations" he stopped breathing. The staff immediately rang for an emergency ambulance while I grabbed the oxygen, bag and mask. His airway was clear and so I tipped his head back and fitted the mask over his mouth and nose, a technique I had carried out many times on a dummy but, luckily, it is not a common procedure in real life. His chest moved as I squeezed the bag. After a few minutes I heard the welcome sound of an ambulance siren. As the paramedics arrived, I took off the mask. His chest moved. He was now breathing on his own.

The ambulance crew lifted him onto their stretcher and went through the back entrance of the custody centre and into the waiting ambulance. With blue lights flashing and sirens blasting out, they were off.

Later in the evening, I was called to Torbay Hospital, to take a blood sample from a driver who might have been drinking. I asked the duty sister about my earlier patient and was told that he was still unconscious but recovering.

"No", she said, "he had not stopped breathing. He is just another drunk, wasting our time". Did she realise that, every year, in the UK, there are ten times as many deaths from alcohol as all the illegal drugs combined? In an eleven-year study, the Independent Police Complaints Commission found drink or drugs implicated in over seventy per cent of deaths in the cells. I was right to be worried; we nearly had another one. Alcohol is dangerous, especially in custody. I was more concerned about the drunks in the cells than the drug addicts.

Why had he stopped breathing? In the base of the brain is an area called the "respiratory centre." Throughout the day and night we do not need to think about breathing; the respiratory centre is on autopilot. But alcohol, along with other drugs such as heroin, inhibits this centre; too much alcohol and the respiratory centre simply switches off.

This is not the only way alcohol kills. Before the breathing stops the cough reflex is inhibited. A drunk may vomit, inhale and, without an effective cough, choke to death. This was the cause of death of the guitarist Jimmy Hendrix; although he had combined alcohol with a large dose of "Vesparax", which contains a mixture of barbiturates and a sedating antihistamine.

I did not know the blood alcohol level of the man in custody but it was probably about 300 mgs/100 mls blood.

When the blood level is less than 50 mgs/100 mls, people are more talkative but there is little outward effect, although reactions are affected making driving dangerous.

At 50 to 100 mgs/100 mgs people feel euphoric. There is some loss of concentration and there may be slurred speech. There can be bravado – Dutch courage and some difficulty in spatial perception

The drink drive limit is 80 mg in 100 mls of blood.

Between 100 and 150 mgs there is a serious lack of concentration, marked loss of perception and emotional instability. It is the drunk who bursts into tears or tells the bar maid that his wife does not understand him.

Once the blood level reaches 150 – 200mgs/100 mls someone would be disorientated, confused and dizzy. There is reduced pain sense that is why, before anaesthetics surgeons used alcohol to reduce pain. When I worked in an A&E department as a student I saw a very drunk man who had cut his hand. I followed my training, injected local anaesthetic and used a pin to assess whether the anaesthetic was working. "Do you feel this?" I asked.

"I wouldn't notice if you cut my f**ing arm off," came the reply.

At between 200-300mgs people fall into a stupor, can vomit and be incontinent of both urine and faeces.

Beyond 300 mgs to 450 mgs they fall into a coma and 450 mgs/100 mgs is not compatible with life. They die, usually from respiratory failure – the respiratory centre stops working.

When the singer and musician Amy Winehouse died, the press and family argued that it could not just be alcohol. It was. Her blood alcohol level was 416 mgs/100 mls.

To make the whole issue even more complicated, the level of alcohol at post mortem may not always reflect the level in life. Decomposition can lead to fermentation, increasing the measured alcohol in the body. The tube train driver in the Moorgate train crash in 1975, in which forty-three people died, was found to have 80 mgs/100 mls alcohol in his blood. It took time to reach his body in the heat of the tunnel and so it is possible that this was a false reading, with the alcohol fermented during decomposition.

Alcohol caused serious problems in custody. Whatever the views of the A&E sister, I knew that we had just had a near miss. Drunks were more likely to be agitated, aggressive, abusive, noisy, disruptive and violent, compared with other detainees and there were hygiene problems, as they vomited in the cell.

Gradually, it became clear that custody was the wrong place for drunks. In 2000 I was sent guidelines stating that drunk and incapable people should not be taken to custody; only drunk and disorderly. However, it was always a difficult dividing line. A particular man was clearly drunk and incapable, not drunk and disorderly but was brought into custody in 2002, two years after the guidance. If he had died, questions would have been asked. But a drunk and disorderly person can slip into a drunk and incapable state.

Alcohol is a depressant; it depresses the stiff upper lip, releasing the real person. This was not a problem if the real person wanted to dance down the street singing but it can lead to violence if the real person is violent.

Torquay is a popular resort for hen parties and stag-dos. This helps the local economy and most behave well, if a little boisterously.

If they did end up in custody, they simply suffered the usual hangover, a combination of dehydration and low blood glucose, leading to a dry mouth and sweating. If sober enough, a glass of a sugary drink might prevent these symptoms. Uncomplicated withdrawal usually occurred after twenty-four hours; with nausea, vomiting, malaise, weakness, depressed mood, irritability, headache and insomnia.

I did see two men from a stag-do who had been in a fight in a pub. Unfortunately one of the men was the groom, the other was the bride's father. Perhaps alcohol had released the real people, real people who harboured violence against each other. I did wonder whether this would be mentioned in the best man's speech. The custody sergeant felt that they would be in enough trouble with the women and so they were not charged.

In my GP practice we had a couple who were both alcoholics. On the rare occasions when they were sober they could be delightful but, when drunk, they rowed. Although the rows sometimes became physical, he appeared to have as many injuries as his wife. Their injuries were never too serious. However, one evening he picked up a knife and stabbed her. She died from her injuries. He was convicted of murder and so the court must have believed that this was not simply a terrible accident.

This fitted in with all the research. Alcohol is associated with sixty to seventy per cent of all homicides. It even affects the victims. A third of victims of homicide were under the influence of alcohol when they were killed. I have no doubt that she was drunk at the time of the murder. It is implicated in half of all violent assaults, three quarters of stabbings and seven out of ten of beatings.

Alcohol is implicated in over half of all rapes and a third of suicides.

Charlie Grey was a delightful elderly man who lived on the streets. He was always apologetic, never violent and he terrified me. He had the classic red face, red palms and tremor of the chronic alcoholic. His liver felt large and craggy. One day he would be found dead; I just hoped that it would not be in a police cell just after I had seen him and declared him fit to be detained. He was at a much higher risk than any of the heroin addicts.

Most of the time he had the symptoms and signs of alcohol: slurred speech, clumsiness and was uninhibited. When examined he had red eyes, nystagumus (the eye flickering to one side), a bounding pulse and increased blood pressure. Alcohol is also a diuretic, which made him pass excessive urine. With the disinhibition, this often led to incontinence.

However, it was not only Charlie's incontinence that worried me. He was kept in a video cell and, after six hours, sometimes had a fit. Although not dangerous in themselves the fits were a sign that he was seriously ill and needed to be admitted to hospital. On one occasion I was called to his cell urgently. He was fitting. I watched him as he stopped while the sergeant rang for an ambulance. When the paramedics arrived they looked at him and said, "He's not had a fit, just drunk." I had to insist that he be admitted. Paramedics are highly qualified and experienced but I had been a doctor for twenty years. I had seen a fit before. The risk of a fit continues for up to two days and so, even when working in prisons, we had to be careful.

Sedative medication is available to stop fits and reduce the symptoms of alcohol withdrawal but it also inhibits respiration, especially when combined with alcohol. I was left with the difficult decision; do I try to prevent a fit by giving medication, when he might stop breathing on the end of my needle, or do I avoid any treatment and allow him to fit?

He always had an irregular heartbeat, alcohol affects the heart muscle. I also knew that the irregular heart can lead to sudden death.

When kept in over one weekend he became disorientated, confused and was suffering hallucinations. Examining him, he had a high temperature, high blood pressure and fast heart rate. He was suffering from Delirium Tremens or DTs. He needed urgent hospital admission. This was serious; one in twenty people with DTs dies.

He was also always confused, with a poor short-term memory. What he couldn't remember he made up, making any interview with the police difficult. Medically this was known as Korsakoff's psychosis.

He survived the nights I was on duty with him but this was luck, not skilful medicine.

When on call as a GP I was once called to an unconscious patient. There were no signs of a head injury or stroke. He reminded me of a patient in a diabetic coma but the family insisted that he was not diabetic. Today I would carry a blood glucose monitor but there were no handy monitors available in the 1980s. I rang for an ambulance but decided that an injection of glucose would do no harm. I gave some intravenous glucose and he immediately woke up. "Thanks doc," he said, "did you give me some IV glucose. It always works."

Talking to the patient, not the family, I discovered that he was an alcoholic and one of the many dangers of alcohol is that it can lower the blood glucose. In a less dramatic way, it also explains the sweating and shivers in a hangover. He did not need to go to hospital.

I was not the first police surgeon to worry about the serious medical problems facing drunks. In 1887 the "Metropolitan Police Surgeons' Association" arranged a lecture on *"The diagnosis of drunkenness."*

Even the police were not immune. Of the first 3,247 police officers recruited in 1829 over half, 1644, were later dismissed; mainly for drunkenness.

In 1878 Dr Francis Ogston, the professor of Forensic Medicine in the University of Aberdeen, presented a paper, entitled "The use and abuse of alcohol", at the Annual meeting of the Aberdeen, Banff and Kincardine Branch of the British Medical Association. It was subsequently published in the British Medical Journal.

"We are only skimming over this social gangrene. The locking-up the drunk and disorderly for a few hours, or bringing them before a magistrate for fine, or temporary imprisonment where the fine is not forthcoming, has proved utterly useless for restraining the drunkard."

Little has changed.

CHAPTER 10
ONE FOR THE POT – CANNABIS

"I wouldn't answer the marijuana questions, you know why? Because I don't want some little kid doing what I tried."

George W. Bush

Lee was brought into custody after attacking a group of men in a local pub. This was not the usual pub brawl. It was a family pub by the harbour. He did not know any of these men, who were just standing together, having a quiet drink. When I saw him he was agitated but was beginning to calm down. He did not appear drunk and was now coherent. He was also feeling embarrassed and ashamed. He had no history of mental illness and was not known to the police; so why had he suddenly attacked a group of strangers?

He told me that he had been outside, in the street, when he rolled up a spliff of skunk weed, the strong cannabis. When smoked it produces an effect, within ten to thirty minutes, which can last up to three hours. Normally, users feel euphoric, although they may have poor co-ordination, clumsiness and slurred speech.

Lee did not feel euphoric. After smoking it, he went into the pub and saw the men at the bar, relaxed and laughing. He "knew" they were laughing at him; they kept looking over in his direction. He felt himself getting angry and finally went over to them. He hit the largest and loudest, who fell backwards off his chair. Quickly the pub staff grabbed him and called the police.

It was safe to keep him in the cells. Occasionally, there can be mild withdrawal symptoms; such as poor sleep and irritability but it is not addictive.

It was unusual to see cannabis users in custody. Most bought their supply with their own hard-earned money. Users normally "chill out" and are less likely to fight or commit other offences than people who drink too much alcohol.

Throughout my time as an FME, I found the police and authorities ambivalent about cannabis. But it is illegal and my argument to the many students who smoke cannabis was that, if caught in possession, they could end up with a criminal conviction. Even a caution is recorded. With most jobs now requiring a criminal records' check it might be a problem, if a previous drug offence turns up. There could even be a problem, in the future, when the student has grown up and has a family. Suddenly, the trip with the kids to Walt Disney World in Florida is a problem. The American authorities may refuse entry to the country if someone has a previous drug-related conviction.

There is another argument that, once someone buys any illegal drug, they are encouraging a dangerous trade; will today's cannabis lead to tomorrow's heroin? The evidence is weak.

It is possible the reason men wear trousers is a result of cannabis. The theory goes that, in about 4000 BC, the Eurasian Steppes' tribesmen tamed wild horses by feeding them on cannabis. Once tamed, it was not possible to ride a horse with clothes wrapped around the legs and so they cut the garment between the legs and sewed them up to make trousers. It is a delightful theory based on very little evidence.

Cannabis has been used for thousands of years and only became illegal in the UK in the 1920s but any attempt to loosen legal restrictions is met with the allegation "soft on drugs" by the popular press.

Along with alcohol and tobacco, it is probably one of the oldest drugs known. Ancient Arabian, Persian and Sanscrit writers commented that smoking the dry leaves mixed with tobacco produces an intoxicating effect. The chroniclers of the crusades also mention cannabis, which was widely used by the local Arabs. And so, in 2009, when Parliament claimed that cannabis was so dangerous that it should stay a class B drug, outside Westminster was a statue of Richard the Lion heart; someone who knew about cannabis and may have even been a user.

Cannabis was a popular medicine with Victorian doctors but fell into decline once the hypodermic syringe was developed. It is not soluble in water so it can't be injected. However it was always an effective painkiller and Queen Victoria was given it for period pain. I bought a "home doctor" book from 1890 and found a large section on the benefits of cannabis; although the book also claimed that smoking tobacco was "efficacious" for asthma and so it was not always accurate.

The idea that cannabis should be illegal only came in following an international conference in 1925 when an Egyptian doctor

A Police Surgeon's Lot

made some outlandish claims over its dangers. His view was supported by the American delegate and so, in 1928, cannabis was banned in Britain as a recreational drug.

It was still used by doctors. When a Cornish practice pulled down the old stables to enlarge their surgery they found a large Winchester bottle labelled "Tincture of Cannabis." It was still full but the senior partner's wife poured it away, not wanting it in the house. It is unlikely that there was any active ingredient still present and even less likely that the police would have taken any action.

Gradually, it has become clear that the arguments surrounding cannabis were not, as we would say today, evidence-based and, as the swinging 60s developed, so there was a need to find out whether cannabis was really the dangerous "vice" it had been claimed to be. Was it really the cause of most cases of insanity, as the Egyptian doctor had claimed in 1925?

The Government set up the "Wootton Commission" a Home Office investigation into the effects of cannabis, which reported in 1968. They reported that there was no evidence cannabis use was causing crime, aggression or anti-social behaviour in otherwise normal people. They added that it does not lead to *"conditions of dependence or psychosis requiring medical treatment."*

In the 1980s and 1990s, most cannabis used was the resin, a sticky brown substance scraped from the buds and flowers of cannabis plants. This was known as hashish or just hash. Resin contained between two to eight per cent Tetrahydrocannabinoid or THC, the active drug. Today most people smoke "weed", leaves from the natural plant. The natural plant has THC levels of about three to four per cent that is concentrated in the tips of the leaves. The leaves are also known as grass, dope, or ganja. I needed to know all the different slang words for the different drugs if I was to understand my patients in the cells.

In the 1990s, skunk weed appeared. This was an artificially bred hybrid of two types of cannabis plants rendering a far higher level of THC, up to twenty per cent. This was not as easy to grow and required hydroponic cultivation, indoors and under lights. The plants were grown without soil but in mineral rich material and plenty of water. Our health visitor returned from seeing a baby and commented how the family were keen botanists with a complicated system to grow their indoor plants. My suspicions were confirmed when the police raided the house and arrested the family.

One of the forensic problems was that, although the effect wore off in about three hours, the drug was absorbed into fat and leached out slowly. This meant that the breakdown chemicals from cannabis could be detected for up to thirty days, even though the drug was no longer having any effect. When random drug testing was introduced in prisons, inmates knew that they would be less likely to be caught if they were using heroin or cocaine rather than cannabis.

The Cannon Street rail crash of 1991 killed two people and injured five hundred and twenty four. The driver was not tested for drugs until three days after the accident and was then found to have traces of cannabis in his blood. The public enquiry decided that there was insufficient evidence to suggest that this was the cause of the accident. He may have had a joint at the weekend but it is highly unlikely that it was still having an effect.

Cannabis smoking can cause physical medical problems. Cannabis smoke contains carcinogens and regular use probably increases the risk of lung cancer but, as most users smoke it with tobacco, it is difficult to be certain. It can lead to a reduced sperm count and even infertility as well as affecting the unborn child. In extreme cases, it is possible that heavy cannabis users develop a cannabis psychosis. This is controversial; it is possible that cannabis simply unmasks an underlying mental illness. This was the conclusion of the Wootton Commission. Some people suffering from mental health problems use drugs to self-medicate and take away the emotional pain.

One man suffering from a possible cannabis psychosis believed that he was an American Indian, despite having being born and brought up in Torquay. He went so far as to set up his tipi in what appeared to be a pleasant piece of open grassland overlooking the sea; he may have even believed that it was a part of the North American prairie but with sea views. Unfortunately, it was actually the lawn of a rather large house on the Marine Drive, one of the better and more exclusive parts of Torbay. In the morning the family woke, opened their curtains to see an American Indian in his tipi. He was harmless and their scalps were safe but, understandably, they called the police, not the sheriff.

If cannabis psychosis is real, then it is analogous to alcoholism. Most people who drink alcohol do not become alcoholics but some do and it can ruin lives. It is likely that most cannabis users do not come to harm but some may become "pot heads."

On my GP list I had a couple who were heavy cannabis users and developed a syndrome of long-term apathy, spending time just looking at the walls and chilling out. They lost their jobs and spent so much on cannabis that they could not pay the mortgage. Although I offered help and suggested they see the drug treatment team, their response was to ask me to prescribe cannabis. They could not understand why cannabis was not available on the NHS. I tried to point out that I could not prescribe alcohol to alcoholics either but they could not see the analogy. Eventually their house was repossessed. Some experts deny the existence of this syndrome. Not everyone who loses his or her job and house while chilling out is a heavy cannabis user.

The "war on drugs" did not always help and could even be counterproductive. After several successful raids in South Devon, there was a very temporary reduction in available cannabis on the streets but some of the heavy users of cannabis switched to heroin as an alternative.

The other legal problem was that cannabis grows well in South Devon. One teenager was found selling the leaves in school. His grandmother had a budgerigar. Where she threw out the leftover seeds in her garden, a large cannabis plant appeared. She did not recognise it but her grandson was more street-wise. He asked his grandmother whether he could have the plant. She was delighted. At last her grandson was showing an interest in horticulture.

A farm growing cannabis was discovered just outside Torquay. I knew the owner of the local garden centre who felt guilty. He had helped the owners of the farm to set up with advice and equipment, unaware of their product.

In another case, during a hot, dry summer, an off duty police officer was walking along the coastal path when he noticed that one area was lush green against the dried out earth. Had someone been defying the hosepipe ban? He went to investigate and found well cared for cannabis plants.

It is also grown by some more up market people. A CID officer investigating a serious fraud interviewed an important witness at her home. Sitting in the garden on a hot summer's day, he noticed that cannabis plants surrounded them. He did not wish to ruin the chances of a successful conviction in a serious fraud case by arresting one of the key witnesses but, as a police officer, he felt that he could not ignore the evidence.

When he left for a short lunch break, promising to return in the afternoon, he quietly mentioned to the witness that he recognised the plants and that he did not want to see them again.

In the afternoon the interview continued, surrounded by holes in the garden.

Cannabis appears to excite the popular press but, as the Wootton Report said in 1968, it rarely leads to other crimes.

CHAPTER 11
DOWNERS; FROM OPIUM TO VALIUM

"Your troubled young life, Had made you turn, To a needle of death".

Bert Jansch

Street heroin kills and I have seen several young people whose lives have been ruined by the drug as well as the dead bodies. So what is it?

Heroin in derived from opium, often grown in Afghanistan and transported across Europe.

In the fields, opium poppies are left to flower. When the petals drop off the central seed-pod is scratched and allowed to dry in the sun. A sticky material oozes from the scratches. This is pure opium. It contains twelve per cent morphine, named after the Greek god of dreams, Morpheus.

In 1874 a chemist, C R Alder Wright, managed to play with the morphine molecule to make "diamorphine." This was over twice as powerful as morphine and was such a useful product that when it was marketed by Bayer Pharmaceuticals in 1898 it was seen as a "hero" and so it was given the brand name "Heroin." Until 1910 it was marketed as the non-addictive alternative to morphine. The idea of drug companies giving a misleading sales pitch is not new. Heroin is still a very useful drug, used carefully by professionals. Throughout the 1980s and 1990s I carried it in my medical bag and it was a major part of my treatment for heart attacks.

The call came from a phone box. He did not give his name but the caller told the ambulance service that someone had taken an overdose and gave an address. The address was a bed-sitting room used by the Department of Social Services, about a mile from the call box. When the crew arrived they found the door locked from the inside. The landlady let them in with a pass-key.

Inside was the dead body of a young woman. They called the police, who sealed the room and called me.

I recognised her. She was a nineteen-year-old known heroin user who had recently spent a night in the cells. Her two-year-old daughter was in care. One of the other residents thought he had seen her in the afternoon but was not certain.

The room was sparsely furnished and she was lying face down on the bed. There was no drug taking paraphernalia such as powders, spoons or foil. And there were no tablets or other drugs in the room. There was no suicide note and no dated letters or newspapers indicating how long she had been lying undiscovered.

The television shelf was empty with only an aerial lead but no television.

She was wearing a T-Shirt and jeans and the body was still warm.

At post mortem it was confirmed that she had died from a heroin overdose.

Another drug addict, a male, told the inquest that she had brought some heroin three days before her body was found. He had seen her inject herself several times. In the past she had difficulty finding a vein and had asked a friend to inject for her but this time did not have any difficulty. He had left her asleep in the afternoon and had no concerns about her welfare. He denied being the mystery caller who rang for an ambulance.

We cannot know what really happened but, as she had difficulty finding a vein, it is possible that someone else gave her the fatal injection. It would also explain the 'clearing up' operation, although stealing the television seemed unnecessary, unless she had sold it herself. If she had injected herself alone there would have been drug-taking paraphernalia, such as syringes around. However, if someone else had given her the injection, he could have been guilty of involuntary manslaughter. This is the term given to unlawful killing when there was no intention to commit murder. And, in best "who-dun-it" fashion, why was the door locked from the inside?

What was less of a mystery is why she overdosed. It was probably accidental. Dealers sold heroin in £10 wraps but to increase their profit they "cut" or dilute the powder. They were not concerned for the welfare of their customers and often mixed the drug with baking power but it could be brick dust or even household cleaner. This was what the addicts were injecting.

If it did not kill immediately it could lead to serious infections and long-term health problems. During the 1980s I became aware of a new disease; AIDS, caused by the human immunodeficiency virus or HIV. For some reason HIV did not become common amongst our local intravenous drug users. For them it was hepatitis that was the major worry.

During my training I learnt about hepatitis A, caused by poor hygiene, and B, spread through blood or other body fluids. Hepatitis B was a potential risk to healthcare workers and police. I tried to be first in the queue as soon as a vaccine was developed for hepatitis B. The new vaccine had to be rationed; GPs and most policemen were not given priority. It was argued that neither group dealt with blood or drug addicts. Only the drug squad and specialist doctors were given the vaccine. The committee seemed to have very little understanding of the daily life of a policeman or GP. However, as a police surgeon, I managed to get the vaccine.

Then another hepatitis appeared, initially called 'non A non B hepatitis' but then a brilliant virologist decided to call it 'hepatitis C'. By the end of the 1980s most injecting addicts were positive for hepatitis C. Not only did they pass it on to other users by sharing needles but, in the longer term, they could develop liver failure.

As their lives deteriorated many addicts suffered from malnutrition, all their money was spent on drugs. They became more susceptible to other general infections such as TB and pneumonia and one even died from infective endocarditis, an infection of the heart.

However, what killed immediately was an overdose.

The "wraps" varied from fifteen per cent heroin to forty per cent. If an addict changed dealer they could, unwittingly, be increasing the dose threefold and, just like alcohol, an overdose of heroin can inhibit the respiratory centre. The addict stops breathing.

I suspected that the male addict at the inquest gave her the fatal injection; an accidental overdose. He then made the anonymous call. But he was innocent unless proven guilty. The evidence had not been subjected to cross-examination and a jury of twelve good citizens had not come to a verdict.

When I had seen the deceased addict in the cells a few days earlier she told me that she was "rattling." Unlike in the case of alcohol, sudden withdrawal from heroin is not dangerous. Addicts suffer from goose bumps (cold turkey), a runny nose, nausea, yawning and diarrhoea. The pupils are enlarged and they have a raised blood pressure and a fast pulse. "I'm rattling doc" is the usual comment in the police cells but, objectively, there were few objective signs of withdrawal. She had been in custody for less than six hours and so I had not prescribed anything.

However, I had discussed her drug use. She had started on street drugs at thirteen, mainly "benzos" and speed. Then a dealer had shown her how to "chase the dragon." By putting heroin powder on foil and holding it over a candle she could use a straw to "chase" the smoke, leaving lines on the foil. These lines are supposed to look like a dragon's tail. Initially this gave her a 'hit'; a sudden feeling of intense pleasure. However, she quickly developed tolerance. Higher and higher doses were needed for the same effect. Eventually the effect could be achieved only by injecting directly into a vein. By eighteen she was an intravenous drug user. But she still needed a higher and higher dose to get the same hit. Eventually, the dose, which would kill a non-user, barely had any effect on her.

If she had stopped using, even for a few weeks, her "need" would have fallen. After a successful detoxification programme or time in prison, the high dose, which was once the only way to get a hit, would become an overdose.

In one year, in the 1990s, I saw twelve dead heroin addicts in South Devon and I was only one of five doctors. All were overdose cases; some having changed to a dealer who supplied a higher dose; others had been in prison or rehabilitation and, for them; the high dose previously needed to get a hit had become an overdose.

All these cases were tragic but one stands out in my mind. He had just been released after nine months in prison. He had inherited a quarter of a million pounds. It had all been spent on drugs and he had ended up living in squalor. His dead body was surrounded by filth.

But were these cases typical? A study of heroin deaths in Glasgow in 1992 showed a high male to female ratio (44:18) with the majority occurring near the source of supply. Victims were aged between sixteen and forty-nine. There were only two out of sixty two where heroin was the only drug taken. Benzodiazepines, the group of drugs including diazepam (Valium) and temazepam, were commonly found with heroin. . In fifty six per cent cases a syringe was found on or near the body. My case of the young woman in the locked room was different. It occurred in a woman, no syringe was found nearby and only heroin was found on toxicology. It was still a tragic waste of a young life.

There are other "Opiates", mainly derived from the other drug in opium, codeine. One of the most powerful of these is dihydrocodeine. This is an effective painkiller but is also used by addicts.

One addict in my GP surgery was attempting to get me to prescribe dihydrocodeine. She was already seeing the drug team who were prescribing appropriately. Any prescription from me would have undermined their work and she would probably have ended up on the streets. When I refused she said, "I'll go back to prostitution to get the money and it'll be all your fault." It is the only time that I have been accused of causing prostitution.

The aim of all drug treatment is to start by changing a short-acting drug to a longer acting one. We then gradually reduce the dose. This is where methadone is useful. This is not new. It was developed in 1937 and has the advantage of lasting for more than twenty four hours. It is now usually marketed as a green medicine rather than a tablet which makes it harder to hide and sell on the streets. However, in the 1990s, tablets were still around. I was called to a flat in Torquay where there were two dead young men. They had taken several methadone tablets. If all doctors had forensic experience there would be no prescriptions for methadone tablets.

Chemists could supervise the liquid methadone dose in the shop, in theory stopping it going onto the street but even this was not completely effective. Some addicts would keep it in the mouth and spit it out after leaving the shop before selling it. One of our local chemists kept a supply of polo mints to give to addicts after their methadone. It was not easy keeping the medicine in the mouth and eating a Polo mint.

Methadone did not give the "hit" of heroin but would reduce the withdrawal symptoms. In a properly supervised methadone maintenance programme, it was effective. If, by having methadone daily, the addict could function and stop committing crime why cut the dose?

Unfortunately, as well as reducing withdrawal symptoms it enhances the effect of heroin and so addicts sold methadone on the street. A study in Scotland found that over half of people in police custody who were prescribed methadone in the community admitted that they also used heroin. There were more methadone deaths from people who had never been prescribed it than deaths in legitimate users.

Was there an alternative? In the 1990s the local coroner became so worried about the number of heroin deaths that I was asked to join a committee to look into the problem. On the committee I pointed out that pure pharmaceutical heroin, injected under medical supervision, is a safe drug. Why not give the addicts heroin under medical supervision? This would reduce deaths and reduce crime. Addicts would not need to steal to feed their habit and would not need to buy from dealers. Dealers would go out of business. And dealers were doing more than just selling. Because some of their "customers" died they needed to encourage new "customers." This meant encouraging vulnerable people to "give it a try", often for free. Once hooked, they had another dependant "customer." So by offering heroin on the NHS we might not only help current addicts but prevent new ones from starting. The only other person on the committee who supported my view was the police officer. All the councillors and managers saw this as going "soft on drugs." The two people who saw the effects of heroin at first hand were accused of being "soft". I tried to explain that, if it worked, maybe it would be the right way forward but it was not a policy that would see the councillors re-elected.

There was another group of drugs that, during the 1980s and 1990s, was beginning to become a problem; the benzodiazepines or "benzos" which included Valium and Librium. While the "experts" claimed that they were safe I was seeing people in the cells who were found to be carrying illegal benzos. They clearly had a street value. The drug dealers and addicts were ahead of the experts in realising they enhanced the effects of alcohol and the opiates. Users needed a smaller hit of heroin if they also took a benzo.

In 1941 Leo Sternbech, a Polish Jew, fled the Nazis, helped by his employers, the pharmaceutical company Hoffmann-Le Roche. It was not exactly "The Sound of Music" but his survival had a far larger impact on humanity than a troupe of family singers.

He continued to work for the same company in New Jersey, USA trying to develop safer tranquillizers. In the 1950s, most of the effective tranquillizers and sleeping tablets were barbiturates. These were addictive and dangerous. Ten times the prescribed dose could be fatal.

In 1955, he synthesised a new chemical called chlordiazepoxide. He was not impressed and put it to one side. Two years later, another scientist found some of the powder while cleaning out an old Petri dish He tested it on animals and discovered a powerful tranquillizing effect. In 1960 it was marketed as Librium and, in 1963, they developed diazepam, marketed as Valium.

The company believed that they had found a new group of drugs, which were both safe and non addictive; a new wonder drug, just as cocaine had appeared to be one hundred years earlier.

It may say more about society than the drug but diazepam was incredibly successful. It was the most prescribed drug in America between 1969 and 1982. In 1978 there were over two point three billion tablets sold.

There was evidence that these drugs were addictive very early on but the research was carried out in psychiatric hospitals using very high doses. Surely used in the normal dose in "normal" people there would not be a problem?

There were numerous anecdotes of abuse and addiction, including from my GP practice and the police station but these were dismissed. As in any review of history it is important to put these views in the context of the time. Before the benzodiazepines there were millions of prescriptions of barbiturates. The late 1950s and early 1960s saw a huge increase in suicides from barbiturates, including Marilyn Monroe. Benzodiazepines were far safer in overdose; so safe that the BMA mounted a campaign to phase out barbiturates. Without barbiturates doctors started prescribing benzodiazepines. There was even an advertisement sent to doctors in America with a picture of a dead Marilyn Monroe. The caption read, "She wouldn't have died if she'd taken Mogadon", which was a benzodiazepine sleeping tablet. I doubt that this advert would pass the advertising standards authority today. Very few people suggested that drugs may not be the best way to treat anxiety.

Alarm bells were starting to ring. In 1980, the UK Committee on Review of Medicines pointed out that, if used continuously for between three and fourteen days, they stop working but the committee still suggested that there was little evidence of dependence; although there being little evidence did not mean that it was not true.

In my GP surgery I noticed that some people suffered from withdrawal symptoms when the benzodiazepines were stopped.

However, was this simply because these were anxious people; after all, why were they prescribed it in the first place?

One of the short-acting benzodiazepines, temazepam, was marketed as a sleeping tablet and came as liquid-filled capsules. Addicts were taking out the fluid and injecting it. When tablets were substituted in the 1980s, it was interesting to see which patients were upset. At last it became clear that there was a problem.

In 1990 the UK Committee on the Safety of Medicines and the Royal College of Psychiatrists published guidelines pointing out that the benzodiazepines should only be used for a short time.

Today the British National Formulary, the bible of prescribing for every doctor in the UK, says: *"Although these drugs are sometimes prescribed for stress-related symptoms, unhappiness or minor physical disease their use in such conditions is inappropriate .... treatment should be limited to the lowest possible dose for the lowest possible time."*

Today the benzodiazepines are a Class C drug, except for temazepam and flunitrazepam (Rohypnol). They are used to treat anxiety but they can, rarely, increase aggression. They also carry risks: in the same way that alcohol and heroin suppress breathing, so do the benzos. Sudden withdrawal can also lead to fits.

As a GP I had to be careful. They were the group of drugs most likely to be "blagged". Some practices stopped prescribing them altogether, while we would not prescribe unless we knew the patient and had all the records. When we did prescribe it was for a small amount.

One man I saw in the cells had all his diazepam sorted into bags of ten and was also carrying cash but still claimed they were for his own personal use. Luckily he was not our GP patient.

When I ran clinics in the prisons we never prescribed them, except in accordance with a standard protocol, for a reducing dose to people who had just come in. Even then we had to confirm the prescription with the GP.

I was once telephoned in my GP practice about a patient of mine who had just been sent to prison. "He tells me that you prescribe ten tablets of 10 mgs diazepam a day. Please could you confirm the prescription and the dose?"

I had never prescribed him diazepam. Perhaps he thought it was worth a try.

In the police station detainees may admit to heroin but not tell the doctor or nurse about the benzos. Not everyone suffers withdrawal symptoms, which may be why it took so long for the medical profession to wake up to the risks. Only between twenty to forty per cent of users will suffer withdrawal effects. The problem faced in the Police station is that the doctor or nurse has no idea who is who. And for some long-acting benzos, withdrawal symptoms may not occur until a week after stopping the drug.

The problem with opiates remains static while other drugs go in and out of fashion. The hippie movement of the 1960s would never have accepted heroin and students smoking pot rarely move on to opiates. Street heroin is dangerous and I've seen too many deaths of young people; wasted lives. However, this is a medical problem and I think that it needs to be taken out of the criminal justice system.

CHAPTER 12
MORE HASTE LESS SPEED

"Cocaine habit-forming? Of course not. I ought to know. I've been using it for years."

Tallulah Bankhead

Darren was brought into custody with several officers. He was a known amphetamine user. As he was screaming and hitting out he was taken straight to the cells; no time for a formal interview at the desk. Through the hatch, I could see he was very aggressive with large pupils. If I had been able to examine him he would have had a high blood pressure, raised pulse and raised temperature; the known effects of amphetamine use. But these are also the effects of the hormone adrenaline which is released when an animal is threatened, ready to fight off a predator or run; fight or flight. Both increase the heart rate and blood pressure, enlarge the pupils and open up the blood vessels in the skin. And he was at risk of an irregular heart-beat, that could cause sudden death.

Any attempt to go into the cell for an examination would have been pointless and dangerous.

Amphetamine was often called 'Speed' 'wizz' or even 'Billy' after the cartoon character Billy Wizz. It was the poor man's cocaine, which is why, in the 1980s and 1990s; I saw more amphetamine in Devon than cocaine.

Amphetamine was taken by mouth, smoked, snorted, or injected. Unless injected (when it produces an immediate 'rush'), it worked in about twenty minutes and lasted up to six hours. It is a class B drug when taken by mouth or snorted but class A if prepared for injection.

I also knew Darren as a patient in my GP practice. He was well known to the police as a user and dealer in both amphetamine and anabolic steroids. This time, I was told, the police raided his flat; he had picked up a samurai sword and swung it at the officers. They had retreated but returned with shields and incapacitant spray. In the 1990s this was CS (chemically known as chlorobenzylidene malonitrile) gas.

He had taken a dangerous combination of amphetamine and anabolic steroids.

The following day, I received a phone call from his social worker. She knew me as his GP and did not know I had seen him in custody.

"Poor Darren", she said. "I'm afraid the police were a bit rough with him but then, you know what the Police are like, don't you?"

"No, tell me" I asked.

"Well, he said he agreed to go to the police station but they hit him about on the way".

I explained that, if she had evidence of police brutality, she should go through official channels. If not, it was inappropriate for a professional to make serious allegations on no evidence. I then pointed out that I had seen him in custody. His version of events was not entirely accurate.

As with heroin and the benzos, amphetamine was once a "wonder drug." In an earlier generation, as a GP, I would have prescribed it.

It was discovered in 1887 when scientists were working on ephedrine, a naturally occurring chemical from plants used to treat asthma. But it was useless in asthma cases and ignored, until 1927, when an American scientist swallowed some. It had an amazing effect. It was ephedrine on fast forward, increasing all senses, increasing the heart rate and stopping sleep. "Speed" was born.

In 1932, it was marketed as a Benzedrine inhaler and an antidepressant but its main use was in "pep pills". During the Second World War, it is estimated that over 72 million tablets were used by both the allies and axis soldiers. It was in "purple heart" tablets and helped the night-bombers stay awake as they bombed Germany.

From 1941, Hitler's doctor, Dr Morell gave him a vitamin injection every morning but also slipped in Amphetamine. In this eclectic mixture he included extracts of testes and seminal vesicles from young bulls. This would have included testosterone, a body-building steroid; a similar mixture which had such a disastrous effect on Darren. After 1943, he had a further injection every second afternoon. In 1944, Hitler told Mussolini: "I was completely exhausted and, after his injection, I felt fresh again." Should we then blame Hitler's refusal to admit defeat and many atrocities, at the end of the Second World War, on Hitler's doctor? In fairness, it would have been a brave doctor who said, "Sorry, Adolf, but you can't have another injection. It's not good for you," although he could have added "and the rest of the World."

In 1950, Smith Kline and French marketed "Dexamyl," a mixture of an amphetamine and a barbiturate, a sedative to counteract the "high" from the amphetamine. It was prescribed to the Prime Minister, Anthony Eden, and probably affected his judgement during the Suez crisis. Less than ten years after amphetamine had affected the judgement of Hitler, it might have affected the British Prime Minister; more amphetamine, another war.

We saw an increase in amphetamine use throughout the 1980s and 1990s. It was relatively easy to make in a home laboratory but required a good water supply and stank of cat's urine. This made it a problem in the middle of a housing estate but easy in the countryside by a river. Devon is a rural county and Dartmoor is an idea site for an amphetamine factory; being isolated with fast-flowing streams.

What also made it easy to make was the availability of the raw material. Pseudoephedrine, was marketed as "Sudafed" to dry up colds. Some unscrupulous criminals with a knowledge of chemistry found a way to convert the pseudoepherine to methylamphetamine or "crystal meths". In 2004, the manufacturers of Sudafed changed the active ingredient from pseudoephedrine to phenylephrine. The original pseudoephedrine Sudafed is still available but only from the pharmacist.

As Darren showed so clearly, amphetamine can produce increased energy but also anxiety, irritability and restlessness. One amphetamine user in the police cells complained to me that he could not sleep.

"If you needed sleep why did you take amphetamine?" I asked.

"I didn't know I was going to be nicked, did I?" which I took to be a fair comment.

As with every other street drug, buyers of amphetamine on the streets do not know what they are getting. In 2000, amphetamine seized by customs was about thirteen per cent pure but amphetamine seized by the Police was only about five per cent pure. Dealers "cut" or dilute the supply to increase profits.

Darren also followed a pattern. He would abuse amphetamine for a number of days and then sleep for several days.

Working as a police surgeon made me a more suspicious GP. Teenagers can get moody and depressed but recurrent amphetamine use may also lead to depression. If a Mum brought in her teenage son or daughter I tried to see them alone. They may not want to talk about physical or sexual abuse in front of a parent but they may also be taking ecstasy every weekend.

This was not only a teenage problem. Long term use can lead to intractable depression or even dementia in later life. After the craze of clubbing and ecstasy today will the next generation of doctors see an increase in depression, dementia and suicides in middle age?

Another danger has the long name of rhabdomyosis; which is a condition in which the body is so over active that the muscles break down, release proteins which jam up the kidneys. Death comes from kidney failure.

To add to the difficulties, amphetamines cause the body temperature to rise. I was called to see a body which was starting to decompose; apparently he had been dead for several days. But then I was told that he had been seen the previous day, apparently well and not dead at all. It was a hot summer's day and it was likely that, when he died from the amphetamines, his body temperature was very high. The combination had led to rapid decomposition.

Then there is the condition known as 'excited delirium' when a drug user becomes even more bizarre, with aggression, sweating and can appear to have the strength of several men. They do not even seem to tire. But excited delirium can kill and so someone who is highly aggressive, running down the road, taking off his clothes (as he is too hot) may be ill but, understandably, often ends up in the Police Station. If someone with excited delirium dies the Police can be unfairly blamed for being too violent or even the way the person was restrained.

Ecstasy became a craze in the clubs although it was not a new drug; it was developed in Germany in 1900 but was then only used as a precursor for other drugs. In the 1970s American psychiatrists started using it on patients, even though it was not licensed. One even called it "penicillin for the soul." Gradually, it leaked out of the hospitals and into the clubs.

It enhanced the effects of the music and lights. Clubbers could keep going on ecstasy, although it was not in the minds of Learner and Lowe when they wrote "I could have danced all night". It also leads to spasm of the jaw muscles, which is why some people queuing at clubs chew gum.

Most users were working and spent their own money on ecstasy; a tablet was cheaper than the huge mark-up on alcohol. But some ended up in custody. These people would simply come down and not need any treatment but it was important for the staff to keep them under observation.

Not only did ecstasy users face the same risks as any other amphetamine user but it also inhibited the kidneys. If users drank too much fluid there could be a fluid build-up. Fluid build-up around the brain could be fatal. But, dancing all night with a raised pulse and blood pressure, also led to sweating and fluid loss. It was a fine balance. The clubs did not help by overcharging for water.

There was a club in Torquay which prided itself on having an alcohol ban but, when I drove past and saw the queue, most of the clubbers were chewing, anxious and probably had large pupils. The bouncers at the door were selling more than just tickets.

I then saw the body of a young man who had spent the night at the club, gone home to his flat, where he lived alone and was found dead the following morning. There was only ecstasy found in his body at post mortem. The coroner accepted the evidence that he had died of a sudden cardiac arrhythmia, or irregular heartbeat, induced by the drug.

The club was eventually closed, on the advice of the police, although the owners continued to insist that there were no drugs on their premises.

The popular press argued that ecstasy was lethal; others argued it was completely safe. I suspected that both were wrong but it was difficult to get accurate figures. Even to professionals the dangers of ecstasy were not clear. There were eighteen deaths of young people in England and Wales involving ecstasy between 1995 and 1996 but there were no figures for the numbers using ecstasy safely. These figures could mean one death in every two thousand or one death in fifty thousand first time users; a huge variation.

Most of these ecstasy deaths were in men who were already known to the drug services; most had taken other drugs and so it is not clear whether it was ecstasy that killed them or the other drugs. Only seven per cent had only taken ecstasy. Many were also taking opiates such as heroin. Most deaths were at home but were at party times, New Year, weekends and in the summer.

We were back to the same problem with all street drugs. If the tablet was pure, the dose accurate and taken without any other drug, ecstasy might not have been too dangerous. But that was not the real world. Clubbers had no idea of the dose, where the tablets were made and sometimes used other street drugs at the same time.

Both Darren's and Hitler's aggression were made worse by anabolic steroids, or male hormones, although in Hitler's day they were less pure.

The idea that giving extracts from testicles increases strength has been known for years. In the late nineteenth century doctors prescribed testicular extract but it was not until 1936 that testosterone was isolated.

In my GP practice I gradually became aware of the prevalence of anabolic steroids. As a GP I heard rumours. Some local gyms were offering steroids under the counter. Some young men had raised blood pressure and slightly abnormal liver tests. One man even asked for my opinion.

"My trainer in the gym has offered me steroids. He says they're safe and will help built muscle. What do you think?"

I did not want to sound like a puritan extolling the evils of drink but put the arguments logically and carefully. Physically they could lead to liver problems, circulation problems, raising the blood pressure and risking blood clots. This can lead to strokes or heart attacks. The natural testosterone levels can fall, reducing the sperm count and quality. This also leads to male breasts, acne, and baldness; not quite the macho image his trainer had in mind.

I do not know whether he did take the risk but he had a right to know the consequences. They were never going to be spelled out by his trainer who was selling the steroids.

The ethical point was whether I should have reported it to the police. It would have meant breaking confidentially and losing the trust of my patient but would it have protected the public? I discussed the situation with my partners in the practice, who were also aware of the problem. We all became more vigilant, looking out for the signs in other patients but did not report the gym.

Rumours and occasional anecdotes are not evidence. I did not know how many people were taking steroids. Research was scanty as these drugs were illegal both under the law of the land and the rules of sports' governing bodies.

There was some published evidence, mainly from anonymous surveys. In West Glamorgan thirty eight point eight per cent of men attending a private gym admitted using anabolic steroids. In the West of Scotland the figure was nine point five per cent. In the U.S.A fifty four per cent of body-builders were found to be using anabolic steroids.

There were over one hundred different anabolic steroids available; each modified to increase the effect; whilst lowering side effects. The most well known are all class C drugs. They can be taken orally or injected. There were two common techniques used by body-builders: 'stacking' (taking several different steroids at the same time) or the 'pyramid' (using the same drug in increasing doses).

But, as in Darren's case, they can lead to aggression, paranoia and delusions of grandeur, not good characteristics in a club doorman or a fascist dictator.

To make matters worse, the type of man who wished to become a body-builder was often a 'macho' type. He saw aggression as positive, allowing him to train harder although it could also lead to confusion, sleeplessness, depression and hallucinations.

In the world of body-builders and gyms there are often spurious rumours. To exacerbate the problem the rumours are often accompanied with the comment that either "your doctor's only a GP; he wouldn't know about this" or that there is a conspiracy by the establishment, including doctors, to keep this knowledge away from the public. In the 1990s, there was a false rumour that insulin could build up the muscles. There were cases of hypoglycaemia, or low blood glucose, in people who were not diabetic. The legal status of insulin was changed to prescription only.

The few occasions I did come across cocaine in Devon, it was found in the possession of a wealthy visitor to the area, who had been pulled over for drink-driving. Even this was rare as the wealthy 'yuppies' in the 1980s and 1990s did not often choose Torquay for their holidays. Lines of the white powder on a dinner plate were passed round after up market dinner parties in the South East, as their grandparents might have passed around the Port but it was too expensive for our population.

However, between 1999 and 2006 the price of cocaine fell from £70 a gram to about £35 so it became an "add on" drug. Our heroin addicts found it useful to take cocaine with other drugs to get an even bigger hit. The added problem of crack cocaine was born.

Unlike amphetamine, cocaine has a long history. The plant, Erythroxylum coca, originally came from South America. The native South Americans found that, chewing coca leaves *"filled the hungry, fortified the tired and exhausted and let the unhappy forget their sorrows."* It was so helpful that the Incas believed it was a divine gift which gave rise to the added advantage of giving the Royal family and priests the monopoly. God works in mysterious ways.

In Europe, cocaine was almost ignored until German PhD student, Albert Niemann, isolated cocaine from the coca leaves in 1860.

Initially it did not appear to have any medical use, but then Niemann noticed that it caused numbness of the tongue and realised that it worked as a local anaesthetic so, when you have a filling at the dentist, you can thank a nineteenth century German chemist for not being in agony. A young neurologist from Vienna, by the name of Sigmund Freud, was one of many who continued the research. It rapidly gained popularity, for both medical and recreational use.

It was allegedly used by Sir Arthur Conan Doyle, Jules Verne, Queen Victoria, the Shah of Persia and the US president, Ulysses S Grant.

During the American Civil War, an Atlanta pharmacist, Colonel John Pemberton, was wounded and became one of the many soldiers addicted to morphine. Looking for a cure from morphine addiction, he developed a cocaine wine, which he called "French wine cola", although it had no connection to France. Unfortunately for Colonel Pemberton, Fulton County, Atlanta, passed a prohibition law in 1886. Ever resourceful, he removed the alcohol, renamed it Coca Cola, and claimed that it offered "the virtues of coca without the vices of alcohol". Each bottle contained the equivalent of a line of cocaine.

In the same year, 1886, Robert Louis Stevenson wrote, *The Strange Case of Dr Jekyll and Mr Hyde,* in six days, possibly during a cocaine binge. A careful reading of the story can be seen as a metaphor for the drug addict; turning the respectable Dr Jekyll into the criminal Mr Hyde. One of the recurring themes of this book is how drugs lie behind many crimes.

The city "yuppies" spawned the second cocaine outbreak, in the 1980s and 1990s; the first one having been between 1880 and 1930, when it was seen as a wonder drug. We have no idea why it died out, although it was probably not due to the action of Governments.

In the early 1980s, there was a glut of cocaine in the Caribbean and so prices fell in the USA. To maintain profits, dealers found that, if they put a mixture of cocaine and baking powder in the microwave it turned into "rocks" or crack cocaine. This burnt at a lower temperature than the powder, making it easier to smoke. Crack gave an instant hit, wearing off in twenty minutes, making it extremely addictive. It had the added advantage of being unrecognisable to customs officials. It soon spread across the Atlantic and, by the 1990s, had even reached sleepy Devon.

I only saw LSD a few times on the streets in Devon. It was sold as "tabs", small pieces of paper that were put on the tongue. They usually had a pattern on each tab. Within an hour of placing a tab on the tongue, the hallucinations start, described in detail in many of the 1960s records. The Beatles' *Lucy in the Sky with Diamonds* sounds as though it is describing an LSD trip; although this was denied by John Lennon.

LSD also produced flashbacks. Once someone had taken LSD, it was possible to have another trip without a further dose. It could be a problem if pink elephants appeared floating along the carriageway when driving on the outside lane of a motorway. My brother, a police officer in London, had to deal with the results of a man who took LSD and jumped through an upstairs glass window believing he could fly. Despite claims that LSD allowed people to gain deeper insights into the meaning of life, anyone who believes they can fly is not showing deep insights; they are hallucinating.

Despite the hippie culture, the hallucinogenic drugs were not invented in the 1960s. In France, in 1095, the French King and his nobles had to make a decision. Would they agree to Pope Urban II's request to join the crusades to the Holy Land and drive out the Muslims? Before the meeting, there was a shower of meteorites and a lunar eclipse. A priest saw two knights fighting in the air, one with a cross on his clothes. Others saw a city in the air. At the same time some crusaders felt the burning of the cross. This was all clearly a sign from God. There was no choice. God had made his view pretty obvious.

However, there was another explanation. It was not divine intervention but "St Antony's Fire" or ergot poisoning.

Ergot is a fungus that grows on rye and can produce severe circulation problems, causing a burning feeling in the hands and feet. It can even lead to gangrene. But it can also produce hallucinations and psychosis. Ergot poisoning could have led to the witch trials in the seventieth century and even the famous Salem trials in Massachusetts 1690s. The "witches magic" could have been hallucinations.

The active ingredient of ergot is ergotamine and, in 1938, Albert Hofmann manufactured LSD from ergotamine.

The pharmaceutical company Sandoz marketed it in 1947, to treat a variety of mental illnesses. It was even looked at by the CIA, as an agent of mind control. By the 1960s, it was widely used by the hippy generation. It was believed that the hallucinations gave a deeper insight into life, the universe and everything and so, nine centuries after the Crusades some people still did not accept that these were just hallucinations.

The liberty cap mushroom grows well in South Devon. When dried out it produces psilocyin; another drug which can produce hallucinations. It is normally eaten and the main danger was not in the drug itself but in the fact people can be poor botanists and end up eating poisonous toadstools.

It used to be complicated. Mushrooms were legal in their natural state but illegal if "dried by human hand". Then the Drugs Act 2005 banned all magic mushrooms.

Ketamine was rarely seen in Devon in the 1990s, but recently made an appearance. It was originally an anaesthetic used for horses but is now on the streets nicknamed special K. It is bought as capsules. Tablets, crystals or powder and can be swallowed or injected.

It gives a cocaine-type "rush" and hallucinations. Just like amphetamine, it can produce aggression and agitation. It was finally made illegal and classified as a Class C drug in 2006.

Every time I open a popular "red top" newspaper there is another apocalyptic story about yet another legal high. "Something must be done." It is impossible to keep up with every new chemical which may, or may not, have an effect. Sometimes, rumours flew around, spread through the internet and through "head-shops". After extolling the virtues of the drug, most websites then put, in small writing, "not for human consumption". It is like selling a baseball bat to a violent psychopath and then saying "only use for baseball." But many of these rumours were nonsense. It was even believed by some that the plant food "Baby Bio" or the cleaner "Shake 'n Vac" had hallucinatory powers. But occasionally new chemicals appear which may have an effect.

In 2015 the "Psychoactive and Substances Act" banned the production, distribution and supply of "legal highs," but it was difficult to define a legal high, or now an illegal high. An expert panel was set up which defined these psychoactive substances as chemicals which *"stimulate, or depress the central nervous system, or cause a state of dependence; have a comparable level of potential harm to internationally controlled drugs"*. The problem with this definition is that it would include caffeine, alcohol and tobacco and so these were specifically excluded under the law. This has removed the high street "head shops" but, as we have seen with other drugs, the law is not always the best way to treat the medical problem of street drugs. By excluding the drugs of alcohol, caffeine and tobacco it has been argued that the older generation are keeping their drugs but banning the drugs used by the kids, although no one is suggesting a ban on caffeine, alcohol or tobacco. The Americans tried an alcohol ban in the 1920s which lead to serious violence and Al Capone. We need to discover why people need the high and treat drugs as a medical problem not a legal one.

In the nineteenth and into the twentieth century, cocaine was a "safe, wonder drug." In the 1960s and 1970s, the benzodiazepines were safe, wonder drugs. In the 1960s even LSD was seen as safe, giving a deeper insight into the human condition. The message must be that, whenever there is a new, safe, wonder drug, be very careful. If a drug has any effect on the body it will also have dangers and side effects. These may be acceptable. It is worth suffering side effects if the drug cures cancer but not as a cure to the normal trials of life.

CHAPTER 13
NOTHING BUT THE TRUTH.

*"Whether you're an honest man or whether you're a thief
Depends on whose solicitor has given me my brief".*

W S Gilbert Utopia Limited.

In what I shall call the "Tomato Ketchup" case I was asked to give an opinion on photographs of injuries caused by a smashed, glass tomato ketchup bottle. I had not seen the injuries before and was not involved at the time.

This was unusual. In most cases where I was a witness I had been personally involved in the investigation and could give my observations. Any statement or evidence in court concentrated on what I had seen and done at the time. This made me a professional witness, technically a "witness as to fact" although, as a forensic doctor, I was also expected to comment on the evidence.

However, in this case, I was an "expert" witness. Not only was I paid more but also I had only seen photos. I was not directly involved but was called to interpret and give an opinion. At what stage I would become an expert witness if I had seen the victim or accused was controversial. A simple comment about how a graze might have occurred does not make the doctor an expert.

In the Crown Court the defence team had briefed another expert whose opinion was probably going to contradict mine. Unfortunately, a previous witness took longer than expected and it looked as though the case was going to continue for several more days. Both doctors had only arranged for one day in court and would find it difficult to cancel our engagements for the rest of the week. Although the court could have insisted, the judge could see our problem. He suggested that, rather than undergo cross examination separately, the doctors could meet in confidence and produce a joint statement.

The meeting was short. I explained my interpretation and my colleague agreed that it was reasonable. He put his side and I accepted that this was also reasonable. We then wrote a joint report that described both interpretations as reasonable. I am sure that this did not help the court which wanted a dogmatic opinion but medical evidence is rarely as clear cut as lawyers would wish.

When I started as a police surgeon courts revered "experts." Simply being a professor was enough to have all the evidence accepted.

At medical school we had a series of lectures from the pathologist Professor Donald Teare. In court a point he had made was challenged. The defence barrister picked up a classic text book and read out a passage. It suggested the opposite interpretation from Professor Teare's.

"What edition do you have?" Professor Teare asked.

It turned out that the barrister was reading from an old edition.

"I think you'll find it's changed in the latest edition," he said.

The following day the barrister arrived with the latest edition. It still contradicted the Professor's opinion.

"Yes, I saw that," he said. "I've had a word with the author and he promises to change it for the next edition."

Now, even a modern Donald Teare may not be so successful. Expert witnesses are expected to quote references and research from peer-reviewed journals. Doctors have developed evidence-based medicine and courts have picked up the idea.

Courts have also learnt that not all 'experts' are really experts.

Some doctors were prepared to be an "expert" on any subject provided the fee was high enough. In one case a judge noticed that the "expert" had also appeared before him as an "expert" in an entirely different case.

"Just what are you an expert in, doctor?" The judge asked.

"I'm an expert in giving evidence in court, your Honour."

And the expertise must be relevant. A consultant gynaecologist was called to give evidence in a rape case. He may have been an expert in gynaecology but knew nothing about sexual offences.

Today there is an expert witness group who oversee expert witnesses and ensure that they are qualified. Courts are not impressed by anyone who claims to be an expert without relevant qualifications and experience.

Despite the image from television courtroom dramas, most criminal cases are heard in magistrates' courts, with no jury and with cross examination by solicitors, not barristers. Basically, the more serious cases, which go to a judge and jury at the Crown Court, are called "indictable" offences and the magistrates' court cases are "summary".

However, whichever court I was in, I had to be careful to follow basic rules.

A young, professional man sniffed some cocaine, got into his sports car and drove through a fence into a front garden.

He looked unwell and so I was asked to see him to assess whether he was fit to be detained. I wrote detailed medical notes and explained that, although anything he said was confidential I would have to repeat it if ordered by a court. I also recorded this warning in my records.

I kept my medical notes at home, although today that would be considered poor practice. They need to be kept secure.

In the custody records, which were available to the police, I wrote "own notes written" so that the defence or the court would know that I had separate medical records.

When I first saw him, the police did not know about the cocaine and had thought that perhaps he had a blackout. However, after my first examination, the police found cocaine in his car and so they asked me to see him again to assess whether he was driving under the influence of drugs.

I carried out the full assessment using the standard drugs' and driving proforma. There was evidence that he was driving while impaired through drink or drugs and so I took a blood sample and he was charged.

In the witness box the prosecution solicitor asked me about my first examination. The defence lawyer, who had only read the police custody record, leapt up, "I had no idea the doctor had other notes. He has been withholding evidence."

"If you look at the custody record you will see that I recorded "own notes written" referring to these records." I commented. I did not have the custody records and hoped that this was true. Was this the one time I had forgotten it? Luckily it was there.

"Could we see your notes, doctor?" the prosecution lawyer asked.

Now I faced another problem. This first consultation was in confidence. I looked at the magistrate.

"These notes were written in confidence. Is the court ordering me to release them?" If I had simply answered a question during cross-examination I would be breaching confidence. I had explained to the accused that I would have to disclose confidential information if ordered by a court but "ordered by a court" does not mean in cross examination. It would have to be a direct order from the judge or magistrate.

The magistrate said. "Yes doctor. The court is ordering you to release these records." It was the answer I wanted. The records were photocopied and, as they were all written in long hand they were largely illegible, I am not sure whether the lawyers could read a word.

Eventually I gave my findings and these, along with a positive blood test for cocaine, meant that he was convicted.

Appearing in court without a basic understanding of our legal system is like playing football without understanding the rules. However fit and however well you can kick a ball, without understanding that you have to get the ball into the goal, you cannot play football. When I started as a police surgeon, the criminal justice system appeared to make no sense at all until I discovered a few simple concepts.

It may sound strange but, when someone is the victim of a crime, such as an assault with a tomato ketchup bottle, burglary or even rape, legally the crime is committed against the Crown not the individual. In a modern, constitutional monarchy, the Crown means the Queen in parliament, representing everyone. We are literally "all in this together". So, if someone burgles my house the whole state is offended not just me. The Court case is not between me and the burglar; it is the Crown versus Burglar. We have an adversarial system; closer to a medieval joust than a debate. Just as the medieval horseman attempted to find a chink in his opponent's armour and knock him off his horse, so one side is attempting to find a chink in the other side's argument. Only one side can win and victory is total; the defendant is either guilty or not guilty. In the English system, however, the prosecution has a duty to act as a minister of justice, to ensure that defendants are treated fairly and no one must intentionally mislead the court. They are not trying to reach a compromise, which is why the joint report on the injuries resulting from use of a tomato ketchup bottle as a weapon was not popular, even if it was accurate.

The presumption of innocence is an ancient concept that has now been adopted in every developed state around the world.

In criminal law the prosecution has to prove "beyond reasonable doubt", which is interpreted to mean "satisfied so that you are sure" – as sure as you would need to be about making an important decision in your own life, before you made it. The defence team do not need to prove their client to be innocent; just to introduce "reasonable doubt." However, this principle has recently been whittled away to some extent by the removal of the right to silence on arrest; the increasing admissibility of hearsay evidence and even certain evidence that the defendant has committed similar crimes before.

Fairly soon after I began my career, I realised that a court is a theatre. Lawyers try to impress, not through great legal argument but by the impression they give to the jury or magistrates. The jury does not decide purely on the evidence. The whole performance is important.

A lawyer who developed some of these techniques at the end of the nineteenth century was Sir Edward Marshall Hall QC. He may not have been a great expert on law but he was a great court orator and this was important. If his clients were found guilty of murder, they were sent to the gallows.

Just as a witness was about to give evidence that might harm his case, he knocked over a carafe of water. Another trick was to blow his nose loudly to distract attention from a hostile witness. Also remember the dramatic way in which he defended the prostitute Marie Hermann.

A doctor has an image with the public. If I had turned up in jeans and T-shirt my evidence would not be as credible to a jury as if I had worn a suit. There was even a drink-driving case when the doctor did turn up to the court in T-shirt and jeans. The defence claimed that the accused refused to give blood, as he did not believe the man was a doctor. Looking at the doctor giving evidence, the court agreed and dismissed the case.

Appearing in court as a witness could be a frightening experience but there were a few games, which it was helpful to understand.

A useful trick was to stand with feet pointing between the Judge and the Jury. This avoided getting into a discussion purely with a barrister. I answered the questions facing the Judge.

The barrister may have recently read up the forensic medicine behind a case but, however hard they worked, no barrister can have the depth of medical knowledge of an experienced doctor. But, unlike a doctor, they are in their natural environment.

Despite the efforts of the popular press the medical profession is still respected; nurses are "angels" and doctors are caring. Humiliating a medical professional could prove an own goal for a lawyer. But the defence only has to introduce reasonable doubt, not prove innocence. How can he or she introduce this doubt?

The medical professional is not on the jury. As a witness, we have not heard the whole story and our role is not to get "the criminal convicted" or get an "innocent person off". In emotional cases, such as serious assault or rape, it is easy to feel anger; feel he must get convicted. But everyone is innocent until proven guilty. There are two sides to every story.

Medical schools do not teach forensic medicine. One case collapsed because an inexperienced doctor, who was angry after seeing a victim, said in court: "it was obvious that she had been raped."

"How," the defence argued, "could she possibly have known whether the victim consented? This doctor is so inexperienced in this field that she did not even know the legal definition of rape. How can we trust her other evidence?"

Over-egging the pudding can undermine the real evidence; so, keeping a cool head is crucial. In one case, a drunk threw a beer glass at a barman. He had a minor injury but was determined to see the accused convicted. He "over-egged the pudding", claiming that the glass was thrown at close quarters. The defence barrister picked up a handled beer glass.

"Is this the type of glass he threw?"

"Yes."

"And how far away was he?"

"About three feet."

The barrister stood about three feet from the witness.

"About here?"

"Yes."

"And it hit you?"

"Yes, in the face."

"And what injury did you receive?"

The witness pointed to a small graze.

"I put it to you that if a heavy beer glass, like this one, hit you from three feet you would have suffered far more severe injuries."

The jury agreed and the man was acquitted.

There were several commonly used techniques when cross examining doctors. If the doctor were young, the barrister would undermine the evidence by implying that they are caring and trying hard but inexperienced. This was especially effective when dealing with an arrogant, junior doctor. First of all, play to their self esteem. "In all your experience, doctor..." Some will be pulled into giving an expert opinion, some will talk. After falling for the flattery and giving an "expert" opinion, the barrister would then issue the killer blow, "So how long have you been working in the A&E department?"

"Two weeks."

As I became more experienced, I also became older. This gave the lawyer a chance to imply, especially during summing up, "a delightful, caring, old fashioned GP; means well but he's been a GP, in the backwater of South Devon for thirty years. Can we really expect him to be up to date with the intricacies of the case?" Again, doubt was introduced.

Another technique was to push me into an area where I was not an expert and then undermine my credibility. The barrister will have read up the research and try flattery attempting to push me into giving an opinion for which I was not qualified. The barrister would then come in with "but surely you've heard for the research by Professor X who said....."

Luckily I knew this game. In a rape case the defence barrister asked me about the management of the specimens in the forensic laboratories. I explained that this is out of my field.

"But surely, you're a very experienced forensic doctor. You hold the Diploma of Medical Jurisprudence and you are a Fellow of the Royal College of General Practitioners. You must have an opinion." I am not impressed by flattery. This was still out of my field. When he asked the same question a third time the judge intervened.

"The doctor has already explained that this is out of his field. Do you intend to persist in this line of questioning?"

"No, your honour" he said sitting down.

Put succinctly I had to: Dress up, Turn up, Stand up, Speak up and Shut up.

What happened if the barrister asked a "yes or no" question for which there is no "yes or no" answer? I was an "expert", not there to take sides but to help the court. I did not "eyeball" the barrister but looked at the judge and asked him or her "If I could just help the court by explaining the situation?" No barrister can jump in, interrupt the judge's answer and say "no you can't help the court." The technique has now been adopted by politicians during tough interviews. "If I could just explain to the viewer/listener a little of the background."

Not only is the verdict affected by the subjective impression of a jury, punishment is affected by current politics.

A young man stole a 50p sausage roll. It was not the worst crime since the Great Train Robbery but still an offence. After arrest it was found that he had received a caution for a similar offence four years earlier. There was no evidence that he was a serial thief but, because of his past caution, government-imposed guidelines meant that the sergeant could not give another caution. This time he had to go to court.

The court was reluctant to give a conditional discharge, also due to his past offence. He was given a supervision order. In total, the 50p sausage roll cost the taxpayer about £3000.

After the tragic case of James Bulger, when two children killed a three year old, youth sentencing increased across the board. This young shoplifter received a stiffer sentence after the Bulger case than he would have done before, although the facts had no relevance to his case.

There was a popular myth that, unless an offender goes to court, he is "let off." However, for many minor offences, the experience of being caught and even spending a short time in a Police cell is traumatic.

Despite the games played in court, often the verdict of the jury was unexpected, although I had only heard a part of the evidence.

In May 1998 a 52 year old man, James Green, killed his wife. She was found with seventeen hammer blows to her head at their home on Dartmoor.

He had been a successful businessman, running a number of gift shops, until his company went into liquidation. To cope, he "self medicated" with amphetamine, cannabis and ecstasy. He then became violent, the marriage broke up and she left him. The house was being repossessed and, on the day of the murder, she returned to help with packing. Their son returned home to find his mother's battered body in the bedroom. Mr Green was found by the police hiding in brambles 200 yards away.

He told the police that he had taken between £100 and £200 worth of amphetamine before the killing.

I saw him on the same evening in a cubicle at the Accident and Emergency Department of the local hospital. It was not easy. His medical care had to come first and so I had to keep stopping to allow the hospital doctors to take their history and treat his wounds. We were only closed off by a set of curtains, so anyone in the department could hear me.

I did not want any lawyer in court to suggest that he did not know who I was or that I did not have his consent to examine him and take the samples needed by the police and so I asked him to sign a consent form. This made it clear that I might have to repeat anything he told me if ordered by the court.

The Detective Sergeant also read him the standard caution. He then turned to me and said "it could not harm my defence any more – I've killed my wife". I wrote his exact words down in direct speech.

He then told me that he had taken 72 Nurofen, 12 Anadin', 12 Hedex, "a lot of amphetamine sulphate" some Night Nurse and some weed killer.

In court he pleaded not guilty to murder but guilty of manslaughter while suffering from diminished responsibility. His injures fitted in with the brambles where he had hidden so the court focused on the drugs.

The prosecution asked me what he had said to me after I had warned him that anything he said might be repeated in court. I read from my notes. "It could not harm my defence any more – I've killed my wife".

The defence barrister pushed me. What was the effect of an overdose of ibuprofen, amphetamine and paracetamol?

The jury could not come to an agreement and so there was a retrial and, three months later, I was back at Exeter Crown Court. His comment "I have killed my wife" and the seventeen hammer blows to the head made it clear that he had killed her. The question for the Jury was whether it was murder or whether it was manslaughter.

I was asked the same questions and gave the same answers. He had now been assessed by a psychiatrist, who had diagnosed moderate to severe depression. After eight hours deliberation, the jury returned a unanimous verdict of guilty. He was sentenced to life imprisonment.

No witness should talk to a member of the Jury. This makes sense but, in one case, I was waiting outside the court to give evidence when, at the start of the proceedings, everyone filed out. I could see the barristers from both sides in a huddle discussing a point of law. But they were also looking over at me. What was the difficulty? Had I been struck off the medical register and no one had told me? Eventually both barristers, prosecution and defence, came over to me.

Apparently, when the judge had entered and everyone in the courtroom stood up one of the jurors collapsed and had a fit. The legal point was that, as a witness, should I attend an unconscious, fitting jurywoman? I went into the courtroom. The jury box is not the best place to carry out an examination but she had stopped fitting, although she had been incontinent. I arranged for her admission to hospital. The only female lawyer present, still in her wig and gown, appeared with a bucket and mop to clear up. Gender equality had not reached the legal profession.

The case resumed with eleven good men and women. After I gave my evidence, the judge turned to me and said, "Thank you doctor. Your presence was indeed opportune." I took that as a thank you.

Sometimes I had no idea why I had been called and sometimes even the court did not know.

There had been a "home alone" case. I was called in the night to a house in Torquay. The neighbours were concerned to find the back door open. No adults were around. As the police searched the house they found the attic had been partially converted into a room with floor boards but no stairs, only a ladder with no surrounding barriers. In the attic were two children, aged about six and eight. I called social services and the children were admitted to hospital where they were thoroughly checked.

I was surprised to be called to court. After the preliminaries the prosecution barrister asked, "Was there any water on the floor?" All I could say was that I did not see any but it was a low attic with one small, low energy light bulb. I could not be certain.

"Thank you doctor, no further questions." And that was it. The parents were found not guilty, although I never heard why water on the floor would have been crucial or why they had not simply asked me for a statement. But, again I had not heard all the evidence.

Sitting outside a courtroom can become boring. I had spent a whole day just waiting. The previous evening I carefully read through my evidence and now could not leave the court building in case I was called. I was also losing money. Court expenses were less than the cost of a locum to cover my work in the surgery.

As the day was coming to an end I began to worry. The case had not ended. I would be needed the following day; a day when I had a full surgery booked. As the barristers came out of the courtroom I asked one whether I would be needed. He told me to wait while he consulted his colleague. He then returned.

"It's all right, you won't be needed. You were called in error."

Court is not the place to make jokes. Justice is a serious business but it can also be entertaining, which is why so many dramas from Shakespeare to modern movies and television feature a courtroom.

During legal training, a group of potential solicitors were told that, if they choose a career in criminal law "you won't make as much money as your colleagues but you'll have great anecdotes at dinner parties."

The final decision rests with the jury, not the judge, defence or prosecution. One of the best answers was given by Judge Lord Birkett (1883-1962) after a convicted criminal shouted "as God is my judge – I am innocent". He replied, "He isn't, I am and you're not."

CHAPTER 14
YOU'RE NICKED SON

"If England treats her criminals the way she has treated me, she doesn't deserve to have any."

Oscar Wilde.

Fortunately, murder, rape, sudden death and suicide were only a small proportion of my work. Most routine calls were to assess whether people in police custody were fit to be detained or interviewed. Television cop dramas rarely concentrate on whether the murderer was also diabetic or had heart disease but this work was important. Every detainee has the right to medical care both ethically and legally.

In the 1970s almost every small police station had a few cells. Care was patchy. There were even stories of officers picking up a drunk and leaving him in a field outside the town. The next time he was seen in town he mentioned to the officer, "it's strange. I fell asleep here but when I opened my eyes I saw a cow."

In 1984 everything in England and Wales changed with the Police and Criminal Evidence Act, known to all as PACE. This laid down clear guidelines. It became the bible of custody work. Only some police stations were designated "custody suites". Instead of driving around Devon trying to find obscure, small police stations, nearly all my work was now at Torquay, with occasional forays to Exeter or Plymouth.

Each custody centre was overseen by at least one custody sergeant. Anyone in a police cell had to receive the same level of care as on the NHS, although sometimes the level of care exceeded that of the NHS. I was called out on a Sunday afternoon to see a detainee who insisted on seeing a doctor for his condition of athlete's foot; a service that would not be offered on the NHS.

On arrival at custody the detainee had to be formally booked in. This involved the arresting officer presenting the history to the custody sergeant. It was up to the custody sergeant to decide whether to accept the person into his or her unit.

"He was using foul and abusive language" I once heard an officer explain to the sergeant.

"No I f***ing wasn't" shouted the detainee.

There were now situations when the police had to call a doctor, including if the detainee "*appears to be suffering from physical illness, injury, mental disorder or appears to need clinical attention*", which is a classic "catch-all" phrase. Detainees could also demand to see a doctor. Dumping a drunk in a field was no longer an option.

Detainees who were fit to be detained could need regular assessments, every 15 minutes, 30 minutes or every hour. A drunk in the cells could be at serious risk. Detention officers were asked to assess "three Rs"; Rousability – call their name with a gentle shake – Response to questions – "what is your name", "where do you live", "where are you" and Response to commands – "open your eyes" or "lift one arm."

Detainees have to be treated humanely, although this is hardly new. In 1689 The English Bill of Rights banned *"cruel and unusual punishments"*, which then became the eighth amendment to the US constitution in 1791 and Article 3 in the European Convention on Human Rights.

But what were *"cruel and unusual punishments"* now rephrased as *"inhuman and degrading treatment?"* Although torture usually involves a deliberate act, inhuman and degrading treatment could be a result of failings in the system. Police violence and poor conditions in detention all come under this article. The right is absolute, irrespective of the person's conduct. A detainee may spit or kick but that does not mean the police should exceed reasonable force.

Sleep deprivation or not offering food was considered *"inhuman and degrading"* but so was keeping someone in custody for longer than absolutely necessary. PACE insisted that everyone must be charged or released within twenty four hours, which put more pressure on the system. Sergeants spoke about the "PACE clock" running out.

Solicitors used both arguments. One night there were two alleged burglars in the cells. One solicitor argued that his client should be interviewed immediately so that he was not detained any longer than absolutely necessary. The other argued that his client should be allowed to sleep as sleep deprivation is inhuman and degrading.

In another case I visited a detainee in his cell who threw his sandwich at me. I realised that this was a non verbal message to say that he did not want to see me. I was called back later as he was complaining that he had been in custody for several hours and had not been given anything to eat, contrary to his human rights. He was given another sandwich. Luckily for my reflexes, this time he ate it.

There was an occasion when sandwiches became the subject of corruption in a public office. Sandwiches were available for detainees, even if they then used them as a missile but, if we were hungry at the end of a shift we might eat one. The alternative was to throw them away. We then received a letter from headquarters. Eating sandwiches, which were meant for detainees, constituted "low level corruption." I did wonder whether anywhere else in the world would see their police as corrupt for eating a sandwich.

As a doctor, I had an ethical obligation to point out any breaches of human rights. Luckily these were rare. I saw no evidence consistent with the popular image of police beating up suspects to gain information. I did see detainees attempting to make allegations. One person, on being booked in, was hitting his own hand and shouting "Stop hitting me", until it was pointed out that he was on CCTV.

It was not my role to make judgements. I had to treat every detainee as though they were NHS patients in my surgery. It was only after one of my colleagues assessed an alleged burglar that the custody sergeant told him "Actually, doc, he's the man who burgled your house. We did not tell you before in case his brief thought you might be biased."

Assessing "fit to be detained" was the mainstay of the work. Peter Jarvis was a fifty seven year old man from Taunton, fifty miles up the motorway. He looked like a professional, a doctor or a lawyer, rather than our usual clientele. But the CID believed that his respectable appearance hid a darker truth. His non-existent "business propositions" were responsible for several elderly couples losing their life savings. He also claimed to suffer from heart disease. Was this another one of his ploys, this time to get out of custody and into hospital? But the law was clear. Anyone should see a doctor if a detainee "claims to need medication relating to a heart condition."

The CID, waiting to interview him, were annoyed. This "bureaucracy" had delayed their investigation. They had met his victims and knew the misery he had caused. But the custody sergeant was adamant; he must see a doctor. If the sergeant had been less insistent the defence solicitor might have stepped in. Alternatively, his solicitor might wait until after the interview and then argue in court that any evidence from the interview was inadmissible. Without letting him see a healthcare professional the police would have been breaking the law, meaning that he was illegally detained.

The custody sergeant gave me a quick briefing. I did not need to know any of the allegations unless it directly affected the examination. It was important to know whether he had been restrained with handcuffs or whether a Taser or incapacitating spray had been used. Alleged police violence could come up in court and we needed to make records whether or not there were any injuries. I also needed to know whether there was a history of drug abuse or whether any friends or family had mentioned a medical condition to the police on arrest.

The custody sergeant's briefing needed to be thorough. It may sound unfair but, legally, if I did not know about a medical problem it was the sergeant's fault whether or not I had asked.

Peter Jarvis was not a typical detainee. He had no past convictions, did not abuse drugs and had not been physically restrained by the police.

First of all I needed to make sure that he had agreed to see me and understood my role. In general practice we have "implied consent." If a patient visits a doctor complaining of a sore throat the patient understands that the doctor will look at the throat. Consent to examine the throat is implied by the patient's actions. That does not mean that the patient has given consent to any other examination. If a woman sees a GP with a sore throat and the enthusiastic doctor notices that she is due a cervical smear she has not given consent for an intimate examination. The doctor would need specific consent.

Peter Jarvis had not asked to see me and so there was no implied consent. But he was charming and co-operative.

We did not discuss the allegations, only why I had been called. There was no possibility of accessing the NHS medical notes; computers in the NHS didn't link to each other let alone with police custody suites.

When he was brought down to the medical room, I expected to find a fit man trying to prove that he was ill. Was I another mark for his 'con'? He told me that he was taking digoxin, lisinopril and furosemide; all drugs used to treat heart failure.

He was either an exceptional actor or he was genuinely unwell. He was short of breath and had an irregular pulse of 120/min. His blood pressure was low and his jugular venous pressure, the veins in his neck, raised. I listened to his lungs and heard crepitations; noises from fluid. Clinically he was in heart failure, probably following fast atrial fibrillation. The rhythm control of the heart was damaged making his heart very fast and irregular. All my objective measurement implied that he was genuine.

He was not fit to be detained.

I rang the hospital and arranged admission. The CID weren't happy, probably believing that he had pulled off yet another 'con' trick but I did not want to end up explaining to the coroner why I had failed to admit a seriously ill man, despite my clinical findings. The custody sergeant was relieved.

When I rang the medical registrar later in the day he confirmed that Mr Jarvis was in severe heart failure, following fast atrial fibrillation. He might not have survived a gruelling interview.

However, I saw another man brought in for alleged fraud, who did try to 'con' the system and he nearly succeeded.

I received a phone call from an experienced custody sergeant. "The CID have brought this man in but he shouldn't be here. He is terminally ill and under the local hospice. Could you come in and see him?"

When I arrived I recognised him. He was an NHS patient, registered at my practice. I had seen him several times recently and, as far as I knew, he was remarkably well.

"Hello," I said, "I did not know you were ill. I'm sorry to hear it."

"They must have misunderstood me," he claimed. "I never said I was ill."

He did have some old scars on his abdomen from operations in the past but nothing terminal. I was impressed. He had managed to 'con' an experienced custody sergeant and probably would have 'conned' another doctor. It was unlucky for him that the doctor on call was also his GP.

These fraudsters were not typical of the prisoners I saw in custody. I was usually called for alcohol or drug issues, followed by mental health and minor injuries. There were people with long-term illnesses, such as diabetes or heart disease but they were usually well controlled.

When I sent people to hospital the A&E department did not always agree. In one case, I was concerned about a drunk with a head injury. The local hospital checked him over and sent him back. I rang the A&E sister. Apparently their doctor suggested that he was fit to be detained provided we kept him on close head injury observations. Perhaps he thought that we ran a mini hospital with a team of nurses. The reality was that there were thirty six cells and one doctor on call from home. Close head injury observations includes, amongst other things, examining the pupils with a torch. I explained that, even when I was in the custody suite, it was difficult to see the pupils through the cell video camera. He was sent back to A&E.

Working in custody could be as dramatic and pressurised as any Accident and Emergency department with the added fear that custody does not have the same public image. In A&E if anything goes wrong the nurses were "angels" and doctors tried their best. The public understand the pressures. But no one chooses to be in custody. Anger can lead to allegations of abuse or, at least, of neglect. Any death will be followed by an intense investigation from the Independent Police Complaints Commission and a public hearing in front of the coroner. Any minor breach of PACE will be picked up by a defence team. We may have to explain our actions several months later in court.

One of my busiest nights in custody came when Cardiff City Football Club played Torquay United. Torquay is a family club where police were rarely needed, even at the height of football violence in the 1980s. But Cardiff is a far bigger club and, with a bigger club, come more problems. A small percentage of troublemakers can be a large number if the club has a large fan base.

At the end of the match a group of drunken Cardiff supporters left the ground and formed a line across the main street. Shouting and causing damage they moved down the road, threatening passers-by. If they reached the town centre, on a busy Saturday afternoon, there would be trouble. Police planning had underestimated the potential problems. There were very few police and a large number of drunken, violent supporters. But they had to be stopped.

Although there were only a small number of police officers there were a large number of police vans. With sirens blaring, an armada of police vans, with blackened windows, appeared from side streets in front of the crowd. The supporters started to run in any direction. There was chaos and the police arrested as many as possible. The crowd failed to reach the town centre. What the crowd had not realised was that each van only had one or two officers inside. The dramatic move was a bluff; but it worked.

As they arrived at the custody centre the alcohol was wearing off and several asked to see a doctor. Some made allegations of injuries. I was called and saw sixteen. Most did not conform to the traditional image of a hooligan. Individually they were timid and embarrassed. One was a trainee accountant; terrified that his employer would find out. But he was charged and would have to appear in court the next day. I don't know whether he ever qualified. In a crowd people behave in ways they would not consider when alone. Perhaps underneath our civilized exterior we are all pack animals.

The following week our local paper had a damning editorial suggesting we should never allow such behaviour again. Personally, I was less passionate. I saw sixteen of the fans and was paid per case.

A detainee could refuse to see me. Although I could not touch the patient I could still observe and make notes. A detainee might be shouting abuse at the police and later claim that he was unconscious or did not know they were police officers. My evidence might or might not confirm the detainee's account.

If the patient was unconscious or lacked capacity I had to act in a way which was in the patient's best interests. I should take account of any information I already had about the patient's views. But a patient cannot argue when recovered that they did not want the treatment given if, at the time, it appeared medically to be in their best interests.

The consultation was confidential unless I was ordered to release information by a court or it was in the public interest. The "public interest" was difficult. The classic example for GPs is the uncontrolled epileptic who continues to drive. Although the GP has a duty of confidentiality to the patient he or she also has a duty to the public. The danger of the patient having a fit and mowing down a bus queue outweighs the duty of confidentiality.

This was highlighted in a case in my role as a GP. A patient of mine was also a known burglar who was suspected of burgling our district nurse's home. He had left the area and I knew, through my police work, that they were searching for him.

I then received a form from a GP in the Midlands asking for medical details and giving his new address. Should I tell the police?

I took legal advice. It was in the public interest provided that he was still a risk to the public and that there was no alternative. However, I would also be breaching the confidentiality of my colleague. I was advised to ring the other GP and, if he agreed, to contact a senior police officer. I should also make a clear note in the records including the name of the senior officer. It turned out that the Midlands' GP was also a police surgeon and understood the situation. He agreed. I rang a senior officer only to discover that, whilst I had been making phone calls, the police had found him and he was now in a police station in the Midlands.

The duty of confidentiality even stretched to the names of anyone detained. If anyone rang the police station to see whether their friend or a family member were in the cells, there was a standard answer from the staff. "When someone is detained they are allowed one phone call. I have to tell you that no one here has asked to ring you." Some callers would get annoyed but it was sensible. I knew of one young man who spent the night in custody but was released with no further action. He never told his parents and they still believe that he booked into a bed and breakfast overnight.

Despite working with some disturbed and dangerous people, it was rare to feel personally threatened. The police knew when I might be at risk and advised me to see any potentially dangerous prisoners in the cells with an officer nearby. But people are not always predictable and so the medical room did have a panic button.

Also I did not take risks. If I knew a prisoner might "kick off" if I refused to give him any drugs, I waited until he was walking back to the cells with some detention officers before I broke the bad news.

I was talking to a prisoner in the medical room; he was relaxed and co-operative. Suddenly, the door burst open, in rushed several officers and he was pinned against the wall; not the most conducive situation for a medical consultation. It turned out that someone else in the building had pressed the alarm. As the block had recently been refurbished the staff could not immediately tell who had pressed the button. My worry was not only for my patient but for whoever had pressed the panic button and received no response!

The only time I needed the alarm, I was standing by the door and could not reach it. Whoever designed the medical room had conveniently placed the panic button behind the patient's chair so that I would have to lean past the dangerous prisoner and ask "excuse me, please could you sit forward so that I can press this button?"

I had finished the consultation and had no reason to be concerned. The prisoner had been co-operative and polite but, as I went to the door, he stayed in his seat.

"It's time to go back to the cell" I said. He sat there. "Come on. If you don't move, I'll have to get the staff."

Suddenly he picked up the scales and threw them across the room. They were not aimed at me but smashed against the wall.

The detention officers rushed in and took him back to the cells. I was asked to write a statement and he was charged with criminal damage. I suppose we could call it the scales of justice.

The management of Mr Jarvis was not perfect but would have been very different if he had been detained in another country or at another time in history.

However, had he been fit to be detained, how can we know whether he was about to have a fair interview? He was an intelligent professional but many alleged criminals have problems reading and writing. Many take street drugs. Are the scales of justice balanced or skewed in favour of the police?

CHAPTER 15
ANYTHING YOU SAY

When I use a word,' Humpty Dumpty said in rather a scornful tone, 'it means just what I choose it to mean — neither more nor less."

Lewis Carroll. Alice Through The Looking Glass.

When I started police work in the 1970s, little thought was given to the medical side of police interviews. In the 1930s police had used coercion, threats, bright lights, cold water and occasionally physical violence and, although the more extreme techniques were no longer used, some attitudes remained unchanged. The police "knew" that the suspect was guilty. The attitude was "we know you did it, now confess". This method not only produced false confessions but did not allow the suspect to open up, which could produce new areas of interest to the police. Despite evidence from Swedish research in the 1940s that interviews are more effective if the interviewer gains the trust of a suspect the "we know you did it" type of interview continued in the UK into the 1990s.

This attitude may persist outside liberal, Western Europe. My brother was a detective inspector in London and worked with police officers from a third world country. They could not understand our system. Surely, if you know who committed the crime why can't you bring them in, knock them about a bit and they'll confess. Why all this bureaucracy?

These dangers were highlighted in several serious miscarriages of justice in the UK in the 1970s.

In 1973, seventeen year old Stephen Downing was jailed for the brutal murder of thirty two year old Wendy Sewell. She was attacked at Bakewell Cemetery, beaten with the handle of a pickaxe and sexually assaulted. She was found by Stephen Downing, a cemetery worker, but died two days later without regaining consciousness.

Although Stephen had learning difficulties and could barely read or write the police questioned him for over eight hours without a solicitor. During the interview, the police shook him and pulled his hair to keep him awake. Eventually, he signed a confession. He said later that he was told that if he signed this bit of paper they would let him go home.

The judge told him that he would have to spend at least seventeen years in prison but actually spent twenty seven years as he was "in denial."

There were two appeals, following a campaign by the local paper. At the second Court of Appeal in 2002 Lord Justice Pill pointed out that the court only needed to consider whether the conviction was safe, not whether he was guilty or innocent. He ruled that the original confession in 1973 could not be considered reliable "beyond reasonable doubt" and the conviction was quashed.

In 1975, Stefan Kiszko was jailed for the murder of Lesley Molseed in West Yorkshire. It was alleged that his sperm was found at the scene. It was only after fifteen years that that it was pointed out that he could not produce sperm. In 1975 DNA testing had not yet been developed and, by 1990, the sample found at the scene had been lost and so could not be checked against his DNA. He was released in 1992.

When his case was reviewed it was found that there was clear evidence of mental illness before his arrest; he was hearing voices and believed that people were following him in cars.

Doctors did not come out of the review squeaky clean. The hospital and his psychiatrist produced reports for the court although neither had asked for his consent. The medical report written before the case speculated about his "violence" even though there was no evidence that he was violent. The psychiatrist had assumed he was guilty. To make the situation worse he had no medical assessment after arrest; the police just interviewed him.

In high profile cases the police were under pressure. Everyone assumed that they have "got their man;" collecting evidence and interviewing the suspect was just to prove it. They did not see this as corruption; only ensuring that justice was done.

The pressure was even more intense in terrorist trials. It was probably this pressure that led to the wrongful conviction of the "Guildford four" and "Birmingham five," in relation to two IRA bombing outrages in England in the 1970s. In the case of the Birmingham five there were allegations of twelve hour interviews, deprivation of food and sleep and physical assault. They were not treated as though "innocent until proven guilty".

Underlying these cases was the issue of a fair trial. Under Article 6 of the European Convention on Human Rights everyone has the right to a fair trial. If an accused did not understand what was happening or even understand the allegations, he could not give a good account at interview and this, in turn, would mean that he could not get a fair trial.

It was after these cases that the Police and Criminal Evidence Act, or PACE was passed in 1984. This included the requirement for vulnerable prisoners to see a doctor to assess whether they are "fit to be interviewed"; although the actual phrase "fit to be interviewed" did not appear in the legislation.

Unfortunately, along with all my colleagues, I had no idea what this meant, except that any further Stephen Downing or Stefan Kiszko miscarriages of justice would now be my fault.

It was suggested that we should ensure that a suspect is physically and mentally fit to deal with "investigative interviews". False confession is the second most common cause of wrongful imprisonment; the first most common is mistaken identification.

A psychiatrist would probably argue that we cannot fully assess anyone's competence to undergo a police interview without a team of psychiatrists, taking several hours. At the other end of the scale, a jobbing police surgeon might be tempted to say "he seems OK to me." Between the two extremes lay a reasonable assessment that might lessen the chances of a miscarriage of justice, while also being realistic. Could this assessment be carried out at three in the morning, by a tired doctor, in a custody centre full of drunks who also need to be seen?

The first piece of research into this area in the UK was carried out by Guy Norfolk, a forensic physician in Bristol who, in 1996, surveyed over five hundred police surgeons. Although he found that these assessments accounted for about twenty per cent of the Police surgeons 'workload, three quarters of those surveyed felt that they were unsure how to carry them out. I was in the three quarters. Most of those who wrote comments asked for clear guidance. And the doctors surveyed were members of the Association of Police Surgeons. At the time there were also many GPs who just did the occasional police call and did not join the Association. The survey was carried out amongst the most enthusiastic and experienced police surgeons. If the experienced police surgeons were unsure, how about the ones who just dabbled in the work?

To make the whole issue even more confused the courts and doctors did not always agree. In one case a thirty four year old man, with a known history of schizophrenia, was arrested on suspicion of murder. He was interviewed in the presence of an independent solicitor and a psychiatric social worker who both agreed that he was fit to be interviewed. However, in Court the judge ruled that the interview statements were inadmissible as the doctors failed to take into account that the answers may not be reliable.

Defence lawyers also started to find the concept to "fit to be interviewed" helpful. If a drug addict was refused medication before interview, the lawyer could argue that he was withdrawing and did not understand the significance of his answers. He just wanted to get out and have a fix. If we did prescribe, the argument goes "my client did not know what he was saying, because the drugs he had been given affected his mind." The solution lay, as so often, in good notes.

It was 22.45 hrs on 15 August 1994, when the custody sergeant asked me to see Ashley Stevens. He knew him well; Ashley had problems but the sergeant was not too concerned. "He's OK to interview, isn't he, doc?"

Ashley did have problems; a past history of self harm and possible learning difficulties. Was he now suicidal? Could he give an interview? He was caught driving a car with no insurance, again.

I saw Ashley in the medical room. He looked anxious. Did he really understand what was happening?

He was now thirty. He told me he was born in Torbay Hospital. At school he had been labelled a disruptive child and, for a while, was in a children's home, under the care of social services. He left school with no qualifications and started training as a carpenter; although he soon gave up.

He could read simple sentences and wrote phonetically.

A month before, the Police had found him at the top of a cliff, threatening to jump after a row with his girl friend. They detained him under the Mental Health Act and took him to the local Accident and Emergency Department. The mental health team saw him but he had calmed down and was sent home. On this day, he still said he wanted to die but, when I questioned him in more detail, he had made no plans and I felt that he was not at immediate risk.

He told me that he had been a "pill popper" in the past, taking ecstasy and anything else he could get on the streets, including methadone but that had been ten years before. He had never injected. He was now clean; although did some the occasional cannabis spliff.

He was still prescribed a pain killing tablet containing both paracetamol and codeine and something else he could not remember. He had recently been referred to both the mental health team and the drug team, which did not appear to fit in with his version of events, in claiming that he had been clean for ten years.

He had been here before and had been to prison several times for driving whilst disqualified and once for a ram raid. It was only three weeks before that he had been to court for, again, driving whilst disqualified.

Unlike in the 1980s, I now had clear guidelines. I had to look at both his physical and mental health. Would his physical and mental state affect his ability to understand the "nature and purpose of the interview, the questions asked and understand the significance of the answers"? Could he make rational decisions? The actual diagnosis was irrelevant.

Making the assessment was a tick-box exercise; did he attend a normal school, did he get any qualifications, what jobs had he done since and can he read and write?

There was also a mental health assessment; including an assessment of his general demeanour, mood, speech, whether he suffered delusions, had "overrated ideals" and hallucinations.

This was followed by an assessment of memory. Simply asking about events might not be accurate and so I gave him a fictitious address and asked him to repeat it at the end of the interview. Another test was "serial 7s", asking him to start at one hundred and to count down subtracting seven each time; 93, 86, 79 etc.

If he was not fit to interview, would that mean that he never would be? Someone with dementia or very severe learning difficulties may lack legal capacity and could never understand the situation well enough for a police interview. However, if he were under the influence of drugs, it might be possible to suggest a review in a few hours. An interview might then be possible.

There was a third option, to have an "appropriate adult". The "appropriate adult" was independent of the police and solicitor and could help juveniles, vulnerable people and those with learning difficulties. This is not only for the interview but to help them to understand their rights and the charges. It was up to the custody sergeant whether to call an appropriate adult but I could not ignore the issue.

For juveniles, the appropriate adult was often a parent. In one case, the interview was set up with the boy's mother acting as appropriate adult. It was then discovered that she had allegedly been selling on the goods from his burglaries. It was a family business.

As it turned out, Ashley was fully orientated and understood the allegations and so I decided that he could be interviewed without an appropriate adult.

As I worked alongside the police I gradually became aware of how police interviews mirrored the GP consultation.

Effective police interviewing techniques share many of the same characteristics of effective medical consultations. In the past, both used closed questions, such as: "how long have you had the pain" or "what colour was the car." These increased the anxiety of the patient or suspect, increasing suggestibility and leading to answers which they felt would please the interviewer. The interviewer was in charge, behaving like a parent; with the patient or suspect, being a child.

In the 1960s the Police developed "persuasive interview techniques." Here the interviewer will try to develop a rapport with the suspect, before pointing out the advantages of a confession. The approach may use knowledge of the suspect's cultural background;

for example, if religious, the interviewer might suggest that God would want him to confess. The interviewer might suggest two possibilities, both of which are incriminating, and ask him to choose one. The situation was exacerbated by anxiety and lack of sleep. But this technique carried a real danger of a false confession; especially in people with mental health issues or learning difficulties.

Traditionally, medical consultations (on the one hand) and Police interviews (on the other), had different goals. The doctor was attempting to come to a diagnosis, looking at all the evidence with an open mind. Any new piece of history or physical sign might take the consultation in a new direction. However, until the 1970s, doctors still used a question and answer format; a format which carried the risk of closing down the patient and concentrating on the doctor's agenda. Doctor's' minds were not always as open as they believed. The Police also lacked an open mind often trying to obtain evidence for an established theory to prove guilt beyond reasonable doubt.

As medicine developed, "patient-centred consultations", to use the jargon, the police developed "ethical interviewing techniques", allowing the suspect to open up.

Surprisingly, some of the techniques, for helping the subject relax and open up, were pioneered by the Germans during World War II. Inconsequential information was gathered from captured airmen and logged. An RAF officer who had been shot down would be taken to an interview room. Sitting frightened and determined to only give name, rank and number he waited, perhaps expecting a light in the eyes, while a German with the strong accent, shouted questions. Instead, a relaxed German officer would arrive, speaking perfect English and offer the airman a cigarette. As they both sat back he would start a conversation. "Is old Bill still knocking off the barmaid at the Dog and Duck?" or "Does Jock McLancy still play the bagpipes in the mess and piss everyone off?" Clearly none of this was a state secret. The Airman would relax. "Yea, although the barmaid is also seeing Jimmy Evans," or, "Someone's now smashed his bagpipes." Gradually and skilfully, the interviewer could bring the conversation around to areas of importance.

As a GP, I used a similar technique to gain confidence, starting a consultation with a chat about the family or even the local football club. Although some patients assumed I was an expert on football and asked for my opinion on whether the manager should have played a 4:4:2 or whether a goal had been off-side.

In 1992 the acronym PEACE was coined for police interviews. This technique first involved planning, ensuring that the interview has clear aims and objectives. Details of potential questions and the location and timing of the interview were discussed. The interview started with "E", Engage and explain: explaining the purpose and structure of the interview. The suspect or witness then gives an Account. This should be allowed in their own words. The interviewer needs actively to listen and not interrupt; focusing on the suspect's agenda. Finally, interview must be Closed, ensuring a comfortable end, before the interviewer goes away to Evaluate the interview.

Research, in 1993, looked at the attitude of the police in over one thousand solved cases. At interview, the police were confident that they had the right person in seventy three per cent of cases; which rose to ninety nine per cent where the evidence was strong. What is not clear is how often the police were confident when they were later proved wrong.

Another police technique, also used by doctors, under a different description, is "conversation management". This has three components: the suspect agenda, the police agenda and the challenge. As for the Account in PEACE, the suspect agenda allows the suspect to give a full account of his version of events. In the police agenda, the interviewer will not confront the suspect but ask for clarification. For example, if the suspect described some jewellery, the interview might ask for a more detailed description. In effect the police keep their cards close to their chest. This can either produce information previously unknown to the police or provide evidence which the police are able to check. Finally, in the challenge phase, areas of inconsistency and inaccuracies are pointed out in a calm, controlled way. By leaving this until the end, the suspect will not know the thinking behind the interviewer's ideas, giving less chance that he will bias his answers.

Counselling skills also involve listening and, occasionally, pointing out inconsistencies in the patient's stories. In one extreme case, a GP colleague had been seeing a patient for years and getting nowhere. The patient complained about everything but never made progress. When complaining about her husband she said, "He just sees me as a skivvy; there at his beck and call."

The GP decided to break the deadlock; it would either move her forward or she would leave the practice. "That's right isn't it," he said. "As a wife that's your role." He did not believe it but had deliberately thrown a hand grenade into the room. However, she did not storm out and leave the list. She burst into tears, a series of problems came out and it was the start of her recovery.

While it is important to ask open questions, there are areas in which specific questions have to be asked. Again, this is a balance which must be struck in both medicine and police interviewing. In medicine, a depressed patient needs to talk through their feelings but the doctor also needs to ask specific questions to assess suicide risk for the patient's own safety. For the police, allowing a suspect to discuss an alleged sexual assault is important but they also need specific answers about the victim's consent.

None of these assessments is fool proof but they should, at least, make serious miscarriages of justice less likely. PACE and the twenty first century safeguards should prevent the return of police techniques of the 1930s of: threats, coercion and occasional physical violence.

CHAPTER 16
BORN EVIL?

"The devil incarnate or a misunderstood man"

Tim Rice (Heathcliffe)

Only once have I felt relief after a suicide. I had known Jamie for many years but it was after I had seen him, on one occasion, in the police station cell that his solicitor spoke to me. "When the police searched his house they found a death list – people he was planning to kill. You were on it." I'm not sure whether it was a consolation but so was the solicitor.

Jamie was a large lad with a history of violence. When he first moved to Torquay he met and moved in with a local girl; one of my patients. He seemed a caring partner and, one evening, I even gave him a lift home after surgery. His flat was on my way and it seemed churlish to drive past his estate when he was walking through the rain.

It was after they had a child that his partner realised the dangers. His violent outbursts had put both her and the baby's life at risk. After meetings with the health visitor and social services, she was moved away to a safe house. Jamie reacted as though we had stolen his property. He believed that he had a right to know where "his woman and child" were hiding. There was no sense of love; merely hurt pride.

He was also a prolific offender, not only for violence but also for burglary and shop lifting. His defence had often been to claim that he was mentally ill but several psychiatrists had reviewed him. All had come to the same conclusion; he was fully aware of his actions and understood the consequences. The only psychiatric "label" was a personality disorder and this did not excuse his behaviour.

Eventually, after attempting every possible method to get his partner and child back, he died from an overdose. His mother complained bitterly, in the local paper, how the mental health services and failed her son. She claimed that his violence was not his fault; it was the system. No one had diagnosed his mental health problems but, of course, we had. The mental health team had consistently told him that he had a personality disorder. He did not want to know; he needed a diagnosis to hide behind and use as an excuse for his behaviour.

For over a century, doctors have attempted to understand the minds of dangerous individuals; known colloquially as psychopaths or, medically, as people with antisocial personality disorder. Jamie was a classic example. The books describe such people as being ignorant of the entitlements of others; having lack of empathy and also showing consistent, criminal activity. But, despite the medical label, he had insight and so had to take responsibility for his actions. If his mother thought that his crimes were the result of a treatable, mental illness she was wrong. But Jamie's mother believed the system failed him; that another admission to hospital would have helped.

The first, detailed account of a psychopath was given in 1888 by Dr Thomas Bond, describing the personality behind Jack the Ripper. He suggested that Jack the Ripper was probably "solitary and eccentric in his habits ... likely to be a man without regular occupation but with some small income or pension. He is possibly living among respectable persons who have some knowledge of his character and habits and who may have grounds for suspicion that he is not quite in his mind at times." Today this would be described as offender profiling.

It may sound strange but, superficially, the psychopath is often charming, which is probably why I gave Jamie a lift home. He was plausible and even charismatic.

It is commoner in men who are often intelligent and see themselves as victims, accepting no responsibility for their own, anti-social, behaviour. I once saw a man in the police cells who had carried out a violent assault on his partner but blamed social services. "They promised to send me on an anger management course and never arranged it."

Characteristically, these people act on impulse and show a lack of remorse, shallow emotions, a grandiose sense of self worth and a lack long term goals. They leave a 'chain of chaos' behind them. Most psychiatric units do not want them back.

Their relationships are usually superficial; they have to be dominant and so friendships only last up to about eighteen months and they have an exaggerated opinion of themselves.

Although there is little relationship between a personality disorder and other mental illnesses, these people have an increased risk of substance misuse.

To look at the biology, a threatened animal will either have to fight off a predator or run. Both acts require sudden, increased energy; which means an increase in pulse rate, blood pressure, sweating (to keep cool) and stimulation of the muscles, giving a tremor. This fight or flight response is fired by the autonomic nervous system.

People suffering from anxiety-prone 'neuroses' have an over-aroused autonomic nervous system. Any minor potential transgression creates excessive anxiety symptoms and arousal of the autonomic nervous system. The 'neurotic' personality would never drive at 35 m.p.h. in a 30 m.p.h. limit, without suffering anxiety symptoms; while the psychopath will commit severe, antisocial acts without showing any remorse or any arousal of the autonomic nervous system.

Accordingly, the psychopath needs a higher level of stimulation than most people to fire the autonomic nervous system. Even in childhood, a low pulse in a three year old can be a predictor of a future psychopath. Because they need more stimulation, to fire anxiety and excitement, they are often brave. Hitler won the Iron Cross in the First World War.

It is this need for more stimulation, to generate excitement, which can lead to substance misuse. We all need excitement and stimulation but most people achieve this through work or recreation such as watching films, video games, watching or playing sport or engaging in music. However, the psychopath needs a larger stimulus, which can mean strong street drugs or extreme sports.

Dr Shipman, the GP who proved to be a mass murderer, was charming; patients loved him and they even started a petition when he was arrested. He did not get on well with colleagues, leaving a practice and working single-handedly. He was arrogant, believing that, as a doctor, he was superior to the police officers who interviewed him. He also became addicted to pethidine. In hindsight, he was a typical psychopath.

And psychopaths are not always overt criminals. The same personality traits can lead to a successful career in business. Without mentioning names, there are occasional, high profile scandals, involving top business people, or even the great and the good when, closer inspection, suggests that these "top people" have at least some of the traits of the psychopath.

Why are some people psychopaths? There seem to be three factors; genes, brain structure and childhood abuse.

Is genetic predisposition to psychopathy a natural part of our evolution; giving an advantage in the Darwinian world of natural selection?

At a Darwinian level, the main purpose in life is to ensure that our genes are passed on to the next generation. For the male this means impregnating as many females as possible and ensuring that any children reach adulthood so that they can also reproduce. In an area where natural resources are limited, children are less likely to reach adulthood. The male will need to remain near the female to offer support. Where resources are abundant, children are more likely to reach adulthood and so the male can impregnate females and move on. Therefore, in evolutionary terms, in areas with poor resources, the caring, supportive male has the advantage. Where resources are abundant, the psychopathic personality wins out. And this theory is born out in anthropological research. Psychopathy is more common in primitive tribes, living in areas with abundant natural resources, than in areas with fewer resources.

The need to ensure that his genes are passed on to the next generation has other, tragic, consequences. A male animal will want to ensure that it is his genes and not the genes of another, competitor male that are passed on. This leads to a male helping his own young to survive but not helping, or even killing, the young of others. This behaviour is seen in nature but we also see it in our own species. How often do we hear of a step father committing severe physical abuse on his partner's children?

And so what happens to the next generation, when the genes of a psychopath are passed on? Often, nothing at all but there are also several cases of adopted children, brought up in loving and decent homes, following the destructive behaviour of their biological parents, behaving as psychopaths. Twin studies have also shown antisocial behaviour to be partially inherited.

It is possible that the psychopath may have a structurally different brain. This first clear example of the structure of the brain, affecting behaviour, was noted back in 1848, with the case of Phineas Gage. Building an American railroad, he supervised the blasting of a large boulder. His team chiselled a hole into the rock and poured in gunpowder. Believing that the powder was covered in sand he pushed a three foot, seven inch iron rod into the hole to compact the gunpowder. There was no sand. The rod hit the side of the hole in the rock, set off a spark and the rod flew out of the hole and through Phineas's head, entering in the lower left cheek and exiting at the top. The 6 kg rod was found 25 meters away smeared with blood and brain tissue. Amazingly, he survived, was taken to a local doctor, who treated him with rhubarb and castor oil although I am not sure that this treatment was "evidence based." Within three weeks, he was out of bed and, after a month, walking around the town, every day except Sundays.

His doctor later described how his behaviour had changed. *"He is fitful, irreverent, indulging at times in the grossest profanity (which was not previously his custom), manifesting but little deference for his fellows, impatient of restraint or advice when it conflicts with his of future operations, which are no sooner arranged than they are abandoned in turn for others appearing more feasible".* In short, he had been transformed from a conscientious worker into a psychopath. He never returned to work on the railroad but, after travelling through local towns with his iron bar as a curiosity, he worked as a stage coach driver in Chile before dying during an epileptic fit in California in 1860.

Details were not published until 1869, twenty years later and after Pheneas had died. However these details form the basis of today's understanding of the case.

Until recently, research into the brain consisted of looking at the brains of dead people; cutting them up and trying to work out which part was responsible for which action. By knowing the medical history of the individual and looking at the lesions in the brain, it was possible to piece together some of the basic functions. If we know which parts of the body were affected by a stroke, for example, at post mortem, we can see which parts of the brain are damaged. This was possible for functions such as movements, sensation and speech but difficult when trying to look at behaviour.

Computerised tomography (CT) and magnetic resonance imaging (MRI) scans took our understanding further, looking at the brains of living people but, with modern scans, such as the Positron Emission Tomography (PET) scan, it is now possible to look at the brain in real time; which parts of the brain "light up" at different times. People are given certain tasks, while the brain is being analysed. These techniques are new. By the end of this century there will have been a revolution in our knowledge of the brain. We might understand far more about the functioning of the most complex organ in the body. Psychology will meet neuro-anatomy and neuro-biochemistry.

It is the pre-frontal cortex, at the front of the brain, which appears to exert control over behaviour; our conscience. And there is now clear evidence that damage to this area can lead to antisocial behaviour. Scans of convicted murderers are different from others, with poorly functioning pre-frontal cortices. But can a child be born with a problem with the pre-frontal cortex – or does it develop in time? If psychopaths are born with a poorly functioning pre-frontal cortex, are we back to the idea of original sin?

Although we know that the physical state of the brain can affect behaviour, does it work the other way round? Can behaviour affect the physical state of the brain? Research in London taxi drivers showed that, by the time that they pass "the knowledge" (the test knowing London Streets), their hippocampus has increased in size. This is one of the parts of the brain in which memory in located. So the behaviour of learning the streets of London made a physical difference to the brain.

If getting "the knowledge" increases the hippocampus in taxi drivers, might criminal behaviour reduce the functioning of the pre-frontal cortex? Were these convicted murderers born with poorly functioning pre-frontal cortices or did the brain change as their behaviour deteriorated? Is the behaviour learnt, and then affects brain structure, or are psychopaths born bad?

The environment is also crucial. John Bowlby understood the problems caused by maternal rejection at first hand. Born in 1907, his middle class mother only saw him for an hour a day to avoid "spoiling him". At the age of seven, he was sent to boarding school. This was not unusual. It was a typical middle class English upbringing for the time. Finally he graduated from Cambridge with a psychology degree.

In 1951 he was asked to write a report for the World Health Organization into the effects of separating infants and mothers. The following year, he published an abridged version in a book called "Child care and the growth of love". He looked at forty four juvenile delinquents and compared them to the same number of normal children. Seventeen of the delinquents had been separated from their mother under the age of five, far more than in the "normal" group. He pointed out that, far from adapting to the situation and "behaving well" the quiet child is entering a severe depression, which could lead to difficulties later in life. Although his "attachment theory" mainly applied to children under the age of five, he reasoned that sending older children away must also have an effect.

Other research has shown similar results. We now realise that rejection or abuse, at an early age, is a risk factor and can lead to later criminal behaviour.

Can we analyse why some people end up as criminals? Although there appear to be three risk factors, genes, brain structure and abuse or maternal rejection in early life, not everyone, with one of these risk factors, will end up as a psychopath. It is when the three come together that there can be a deadly result. We can see these factors in well known psychopaths such as Hitler, who had a violent father and suffered rejection as a child.

Until the last few years, there was little effective treatment for personality disorders. They do not believe that they have a problem;

it is the rest of the world which is dysfunctional. The only approach has been to point out that their committing crime is not in their interests. We cannot appeal to the conscience of someone with a poorly functioning pre-frontal cortex or no conscience.

NICE, the body which looks at evidence and advises on medical care has now made some recommendations for the treatment of antisocial personality disorder but these are a little vague.

First of all, NICE suggests, we need to treat any other problems, such as substance misuse.

Therapeutic drugs are also not the answer. Any therapist must build an optimistic and trusting relationship, exploring options, in an open and non judgemental manner. A punitive approach is less likely to be successful. But NICE are less clear on exactly how to approach talking therapy. What does a therapist actually do? They suggest working in groups to address impulsiveness, interpersonal relationships and antisocial behaviour. "Treatment" appears to be in its very early days.

As we begin to understand the criminal mind, so we enter an ethical minefield. One murderer in America turned out to have a cyst pressing on the pre-frontal lobe of the brain. In another American case, a man who started to abuse children in middle age had a brain tumour. When removed, his paedophiliac behaviour stopped; when the tumour recurred, the behaviour returned. Were these two people criminals or were they ill? As we learn more about the criminal mind, will we be able to treat criminality as an "illness." We cannot change the genes or the upbringing but we might be able to mitigate some of the results. Is it ethical to try to change a personality?

CHAPTER 17
ALL CHANGE

"Nowadays people know the price of everything and the value of nothing".

Oscar Wilde *The picture of Dorian Grey.*

Throughout the 1980s and 1990s, there was one Orwellian mantra; "Public bad, private good." Everything, from water to energy; from telephones to trains was to be run by private companies. In 1990, even the NHS changed to embrace an "internal market." GP fundholders were "customers" buying care for their patients from hospitals or "providers".

I was also aware of the bureaucracy involved. In the new health service contract for GPs, I read, *"The contractor has not elected to be regarded as a Health Service body for the purposes of Section 4 of the 1990 Act. Accordingly this contract is not an NHS contract. If the contractor has elected to be regarded as a health service body for the pursuant of section 4 of the 1990 Act pursuant to regulation 10 of the regulations the contract must state that it is an NHS contract."* I was sure that made sense to someone and was important for the medical politicians. Committees probably spent hours on such problems but I was not sure how it helped the patients.

Five self employed police surgeons, on call in south Devon, running our own rota and claiming call out fees, did not fit the Zeitgeist. Where was the private company? Where was the competition? Where was the free market? Other police services from catering to forensic laboratories were "outsourced". Private companies had to bid for contracts. Competitive tendering was imperative. The same approach was taken in the NHS. Cleaning, car parking and even some routine operations were outsourced to private companies. We were dinosaurs. The Police Surgeon service was to be open to competitive tender. Although the system of self employed GPs in their own rota appeared to work well in south Devon, there were stories of colleagues elsewhere, in Devon and Cornwall, abusing the system.

If we saw several detainees, the fee was higher for the first call and slightly less for subsequent cases seen on the same visit. This was reasonable but we heard about a colleague who lived close to the police station, who went home between each case, to claim the higher fee, every time. Others were still receiving a retainer from the police but refusing to visit the police station. Using self-employed police surgeons without a clear contract and payment for each call-out was not working. There was no overall, quality control for our police work. All five doctors working in south Devon were experienced and three had further forensic qualifications but this was not always the case both nationally and locally. We only had additional qualifications because of professional pride not because of competition.

The first rumblings of a change came from the Midlands. A private company which already provided a GP out-of-hours service were awarded the contract to run the clinical, forensic medical services. Initially, the company employed the same doctors to provide the same service but would this always be the case? We reassured ourselves that this was the Midlands; a very different area from Devon and Cornwall. We believed that were safe from being "privatised".

At the same time, there was another movement. In 1992, the Police in Melbourne, Australia, piloted the use of nurses as the first point of contact in custody. Over fifteen months, the nurses carried out over three thousand examinations and the world kept spinning. Feedback from doctors, police and the prison service found the system popular. Interestingly, the researchers do not appear to have asked the "customers"; the prisoners.

Kent Police then ran a trial, using nurses, rather than doctors, for most of the work. Again, this fitted in with the current mood. In the NHS, the role of nurses was expanding. Nurse practitioners were taking over many roles in hospitals, which were previously the province of doctors and it was working. There was no reason why nurses could not carry out work in custody units. The law overseeing custody, specified in the Police and Criminal Evidence Act referred to doctors, in most areas but this was amended. Nurses are better than doctors at following protocols; the service might even improve. However, the underlying belief was that it would save money. Nurses are cheaper than doctors and private companies, in competition for the work, would improve efficiency and bring down costs.

Devon and Cornwall could not buck the trend for ever. In the early 2000s, we heard that they were looking at "outsourcing." We were told that this would make very little difference to the doctors; it was purely administrative. After all, they had successfully outsourced helicopter pilots; so why not doctors?

At the height of the controversy, I was working in the custody centre, when the Chief Inspector, head of custody throughout Devon and Cornwall, said to me "Can I have a quiet word?" We went into the medical room, which was being redecorated. I waited for the important question; had the force made a crucial decision? Did I still have a job in forensic medicine?

"Where do you want the light over the couch?" He asked.

The contract had been awarded to a private, medical locum agency with no experience of clinical forensic medicine. However, they were keen and had exciting plans. Of the five doctors covering South Devon three resigned. The new company did not replace them leaving two of us to carry out the work of five.

Even I was beginning to believe that changes were needed and this might be the catalyst. Sitting and complaining was not going to help. Could this be an opportunity to improve the service?

I was asked by the company, which had been awarded the contract, to help arrange training for their new doctors and give a few lectures.

My work carried on, as before, under the new company, except that the claims for payment were now sent to their head office. They also worked out our rota. And they were reassuring. In an e-mail, I was told that they were "the only provider to pay National rates to its doctors for fees and mileage;" adding "This will not change and I look forward to building stronger relationships with individual clinicians and the AFP (Association of Forensic Physicians) as a whole."

Every year the Association of Forensic Physicians published the new, recommended, national rates for fees and mileage but, for us, every year the fees and rates remained unchanged. This promise was never kept, unless the phrase "this will not change" referred to the actual fees rather than the policy. My contract with the new company did not mention any scale of fees. I had been naive. I did receive a letter, telling me that the nationally agreed rate for mileage was £54 /mile but, sadly, was later told they had put the decimal point in the wrong place.

As they recruited their own doctors, so my shifts were reducing. I was too expensive. They also started employing nurses.

Did it matter if my job with the police was on the line, if the service improved? Although some of their doctors were excellent, some were not. The contract recommended that ten per cent of doctors engaged should have the "Diploma of Medical Jurisprudence", an exam tailored to the work. I was the only one left, engaged by the company in Devon and Cornwall with this diploma –and I was being sidelined.

Stories started appearing in the local media; including one about a police doctor, who had thrown all his notes, about a rape examination, in a public waste-paper bin.

I was now in my fifties and, although I still enjoyed the work, getting out of bed at night was getting harder. Work in the practice was also more intense.

Driving to the police station one night, I stopped at some traffic lights. I then remember waking up to hear the traffic driving passed. I had fallen asleep. I knew that tired driving is as dangerous as drink-driving. If I was so tired, was I making the right decisions for my patients; both in the surgery and the detainees at the police station?

Driving home at 04-00 hrs, after a visit to the custody centre, I was on the outer lane of the dual-carriageway, turning right at the next roundabout, when I saw a fox sitting in the middle of my lane. I swung the steering, misjudging the situation and hit the crash barrier. I managed to steer the car off the road but it was written-off. There were no other cars around and I was not hurt – but was this simply an error of judgement, in attempting to avoid a fox, or was it a symptom of something more? Was I too tired? Was there even a fox; fatigue and light can play tricks in the night? I had to think through my workload. I enjoyed the work and had developed a level of expertise but I did not want to give up the day job, my GP surgery. Police work would always mean getting up at night; burglars, rapists and murderers do not work nine to five.

After three years, the same company won the contract again. It was then that I received a letter saying: "Thank you but we don't need you anymore." I was relieved and disappointed but not surprised. I received a supportive e-mail from a colleague who had also lost his job; suggesting that "*in reality Devon and Cornwall Police are fighting their own battle for survival and we are a side issue.*" Perhaps he was right.

Although standards appeared to be slipping, as budgets were given priority, there was another movement pulling in the opposite direction. Ever since I had started I had been a member of the Association of Police Surgeons, although recently we had changed the name to the Association of Forensic Physicians. They ran regular courses, an annual conference; set standards and published a journal. Now they were set to become an academic body. Under the umbrella of the Royal College of Physicians, the leading forensic medical examiners nationally created the Faculty of Forensic and Legal Medicine and clinical, forensic medicine became recognised as a speciality by the General Medical Council. As standards were being set at

A Police Surgeon's Lot

the top, standards were actually slipping, as police forces outsourced to the cheapest bidder.

There were plans to set an examination, to become a member of the new faculty but I was asked to join under the "grandfather's clause." I was not yet a grandfather but my qualifications and experience were enough. However, I had been sacked by the local police force. I was no longer a forensic physician. I had made a decision to move on. Why should I spend my money to join?

With the philosophy "it was good while it lasted", I moved on. I did wonder whether to approach some defence lawyers. With my knowledge and experience I could probably find loop holes in the work of the new doctors and help some burglars to get away. But I decided to concentrate on General Practice; my day job.

It was about a year after this that I received an e-mail from the police. The private contractor had a few problems but, whenever the police expressed concern, they were told that they were not medically qualified and could not comment on the medical care of patients. Any query was sent to their medical director. The police force needed a doctor, independent from both the police and the company, who could advise. Most of the old "police surgeons", with paper qualifications, had jumped ship, before they were pushed overboard and I had been the last man standing.

The e-mail went on to ask whether I could return, on a three-hours-a-week contract, as the "Independent Clinical Consultant?" It would mean writing protocols, sitting on committees and giving advice. It would not mean seeing patients and, most importantly, it would not mean getting out of bed in the middle of the night. As I was then approaching sixty and the children had left home, this sounded like a good option. I accepted. When I mentioned it to one of my former colleagues, his comment was: "you must be mad."

Budgets were also being squeezed, as the free market was introduced into other areas of forensic medicine. Private forensic laboratories were now being used and the nationalised Forensic Science Service was disbanded. Officers had to balance the need for forensic tests of evidence, against the budget. Most of the samples taken during examinations were never used.

It was not only in forensic medicine that budgets were given priority over solving crime.

Back in 1992, I joined my sister-in-law, at New Scotland Yard, at an award ceremony. It was not for me but for my brother, Arthur. A two year old had been killed by his step-father. As a Detective Inspector, overseeing child protection, Arthur had successfully run the murder enquiry, leading to a conviction. The accused argued that the death followed a one-off violent attack which, tragically, led to the child's death. Arthur, using the intelligence picked up during the investigation and his gut feeling, believed that the child had been the victim of sustained abuse throughout his life. The death was deliberate; murder. The first post-mortem examination found no evidence to support Arthur's theory and so he had ordered another one. Again, there was no evidence of long term abuse. But he was still not convinced and so he arranged a third post mortem, with an acknowledged expert in the field of child abuse. This time he was proved right; there were multiple, subtle clues suggesting sustained abuse over the child's life. The step-father was convicted of murder and the Old Bailey judge commended Arthur's work. But what was even more impressive was that, throughout the investigation, Arthur was dying of cancer. He was not around to receive his commendation at New Scotland Yard.

I was discussing this case recently with a police officer who commented, "It couldn't happen today." This was not because today's officers are any less competent or hard-working than Arthur. Today, I was told, "there's no way a modern force would pay for three post-mortem examinations." Every test must be justified and a gut feeling that the pathologist had got it wrong is not justification. The stepfather would have been convicted of manslaughter and would not have been given a life sentence. Perhaps he might even have been released, to find another partner and to abuse and to kill another child.

The budget for all forensic tests, including post-mortem examinations, is limited. The forensic laboratories are in competition to provide the cheapest service, although they would probably use the phrase "value for money."

Where, then, does the future lie for clinical forensic medicine? The basic work in the police station is now a nurse-led service. The day-to-day, clinical, forensic work in the police stations is carried out by nurses. The move to nurses will probably be extended to the sexual assault referral centres (SARCs) dealing with sexual offences.

The doctors will become consultants, available, as experts, to oversee and advise the nursing team. Their expertise should also be available to police officers, assisting with forensic advice, during an investigation. However, without doctors on the front line, where are these experts going to gain their expertise? While the Faculty of Forensic and Legal Medicine tries to raise standards, the private "providers" try to reduce costs, by employing doctors at the lowest rate possible. The FME needs to become a specialist, with the same status and income, as any other consultant working in the NHS. This will require a career structure with training posts, leading to eventual appointment as a consultant. It will require funding but, in the long run, should prove an important investment.

These changes take place against a background of falling crime. The number of detainees in the custody centres of Devon and Cornwall has nearly halved over the last twenty years.

Clinical forensic medicine needs to look beyond the day-to-day and ask basic questions. Why do people commit crime and can we continue to reduce the levels?

Although every politician tries to take the credit for a reduction in crime, it has been reducing for a thousand years. Despite scare stories in the press and from the right wing politicians, we live in the most peaceful and safe society in human history.

If we look at, arguably, the most serious crime, which is murder, estimations are difficult. In Norman times, at the end of the eleventh century, it was only murder if a foreigner or Frenchman was killed. Killing an Anglo-Saxon Englishman did not count as murder.

Violence, which was once considered normal behaviour, is now illegal and unacceptable. "Spare the rod and spoil the child" is seen today as child abuse. Queen Victoria's daughter, Vicky, was engaged at 14 when her future husband, the heir to the Prussian throne, was 24. Today he would be arrested.

As violent behaviour was normal, so the records are sketchy. The 1278 London Eyre Court recorded about six homicides a year, including two homicides which took place after a game of chess. Modern football violence is tame when compared with medieval chess.

Looking at the population of the time, we can estimate the homicide rate as about fifteen per hundred thousand a year. . This probably dropped to ten per hundred thousand by 1600 and one per hundred thousand, in the twentieth century. Research on homicides in Kent, from 1560 to 1985, showed a continuous, tenfold fall over the four hundred years. Other research has shown a similar fall in violence and murder in Norway, Sweden and the Netherlands.

Although the twentieth century had two appalling world wars and numerous atrocities, such as those perpetrated by the ISIS, the Pol Pot Regime in Cambodia and the Rwandan massacres, when compared with the size of the world's population, many medieval wars were even worse.

The same fall is seen in other violent crime; although this is difficult to measure. These figures may not be accurate. It is possible that, in the Middle Ages and the early modern period, as few as ten per cent of homicides came to court. We do not even know whether this ten per cent were truly homicides in the modern sense.

Today the homicide rate is an accurate reflection of the overall rate of violent crime but was this always the case, in the past? Again we don't know.

Could it be that the reduction in the number of murders is not only due to a reduction in violence but also a reflection of improved medical care? Would some of the victims of murder have survived if taken to a modern A&E department? Any deaths which occurred immediately would still not survive; they would not reach hospital. Again, the figures are not clear but, in seventieth century Castile, about seventy per cent of victims died within the first twenty four hours; with thirty seven per cent being killed immediately. Improved medical care may have a marginal effect on the figures but it is likely that the reduction in murder and violent crime is real.

So why has violent crime and murder reduced? One theory, from the German Sociologist Norbert Elias, suggested that, as the state expanded and people became more economically dependent on each other, so violence decreased. If we are all interdependent for our food, shelter and general well-being, so we need to work together.

Perhaps, then, the real question is: why don't we all commit crime? There are two reasons: external and internal; either fear of the state or an internal belief system. Although politicians talk about being "tough on crime"; increasing the external pressure, the evidence suggests that external pressures are not always predominant in a liberal, democratic state. Two hundred years ago, prisons were appalling; the death penalty was available for over two hundred crimes and over one hundred and sixty thousand people were transported to Australia for such minor crimes as stealing a handkerchief. Today, prisons are far more humane, sentences shorter and, throughout Europe, there is no death penalty. And yet the crime rate has continued to fall. In countries where there is still the death penalty, such as in some states in the USA, the murder rate is high. So the reason we do not commit crime is internal not external. We don't commit crime because an internal voice is telling us it is wrong. This even applies to minor crimes. I could probably get away with shoplifting – but I would have sleepless nights.

In the UK there are almost no provisions for legal homicide. Very rarely, killing might be legal to protect oneself or others from grievous attack or murder but only when there is no alternative.

Contrast this with the penal code of Texas, which makes homicide acceptable when "killing a public enemy, executing a convict, acting to a lawful order from a police officer, preventing escape of someone detained legally, suppressing a riot, preventing the completion of a criminal act, responding by a husband to provocation by an act of adultery, defending a person or property, defending oneself against unlawful attack and defending property rights".

The difference in attitude, between the UK and Texas, is reflected in the fact that, in the UK, about one third of killers commit suicide whilst, in the US it is three to four per cent. This rises to ten per cent in Canada and forty two per cent in Denmark. In the UK the killer had committed a crime which, whatever the motivation, is an abomination; whilst, in the USA many may see his crime as justified?

The evidence is clear; being "tough on crime" does not work. Anyone arrested must be treated with compassion. Of course some criminals need to be detained to protect the public but as we understand more about the causes of crime, learn to treat drug addiction as a medical problem not a legal one and understand the workings and anatomy of the psychopath so we will move into an era when criminal behaviour is seen as deviant behaviour. Deviant behaviour requires treatment not punishment. We must aim to move from the punishment of crime to the treatment of crime. This might make a police surgeon's lot a happy one.

REFERENCES

Chapter 2 Real murder most foul

1. Green M A "Getting away with murder" The Police Surgeon on 41 April 1993 p20
2. Soothill K "Murder: the importance of the structural and cultural conditions of society" The Journal of Clinical Forensic Medicine (1996) 3 161-165
3. Kirk, S "Crime investigation: physical evidence and the police laboratory". Interscience Publishers, Inc.: New York, 1953
4. Petherick, W A,, Turvey B E, Feruson C E "Forensic Criminology 2010. Elsevier Academic Press 2010
5. Bernard Knight. "Legal Aspects of Medical Practice" Churchill Livingstone 1992
6. Steven Karch. "Is post-mortem toxicology quackery?" Journal of Clinical and Forensic Medicine (2003) 10 197-198
7. Provincial Medical Journal and retrospect of the medical sciences

    a. No. 157 LONDON, SATURDAY, SEPT. 30, 1843. PRICE SIXPENCE.

8. Home office statistical bulletin. Crimes detected in England and Wales 2012/13 (Second edition) *Kevin Smith (Editor), Paul Taylor and Meghan Elkin*

Chapter 3 I cannot face tomorrow

9. Depression: Management of depression in primary and secondary care National Clinical Practice Guideline Number 23 NICE
10. A conditional model for estimating the increase in suicides associated with the 2008–2010 economic recession in England Carme Saurina, Basili Bragulat, Marc Saez, Guillem López-Casasnovas - Journal of Epidemiology and Community Health 2013;67:779–787.
11. The history of suicide – SOARS.org
12. Suicide in Puccini's operas. Salib Medicine Science and the Law vol 42, 1 Jan 2002 pp27-29
13. Ministry of Justice "Guide to Coroners and Inquests and Charter for coroner".
14. Assessing risk of suicide or self harm in adults. R. Morriss, N Kapur, R Byng. BMJ 12th October 2013:347 p 33-35

Chapter 4 Mad Bad and Sad

15. The History of Mental Illness: From "Skull Drills" to "Happy Pills" Allison M. Foerschner Student Pulse 2010, VOL. 2 NO. 09
16. A review of Police Custody as a Place of Safety (2008). (Docking, M., Grace, K. and Bucke, T. (2008): *Police Custody as a "Place of Safety": Examining the Use of Section 136 of the Mental Health Act 1983.* IPCC Research and Statistics Series, Paper 11. London: Independent Police Complaints Commission.)

17. Analysis - Healthcare in Prisons - Dealing with mental disorder in prisoners BMJ 2012;345:e7280 (Published 22 November 2012)

Chapter 5 Not like sex at all

18. The epidemiology of drug facilitated sexual assault. Michael Hurley, Helen Parker, David Wells. Journal of Clinical Forensic Medicine. 13 (2006) 181-185
19. "More or less" Radio 4 28/8/09

Chapter 6 I'll drive, I'm too drunk to sing

20. Driving:alcohol Louise Butcher Published House of Commons Library, Standard note SN788, 11 April 2013.
21. Drinking and driving: a decrease in executive frontal functions in young drivers with high blood alcohol concentration" S C A Domingues, J B Mendonca, R Laranjeira. December 2009 Alcohol Vol. 43, Issue 8, Pages 657-664
22. Department for Transport. Reported road casualties in Britain. 2013. www.gov.uk/government/uploads/system/uploads/attachment_data/file/226068/accidents-involving-illegal-alcohol-levels-2011-2012.pdf.
23. Alcohol intoxication in road traffic accidents leads to higher impact speed difference, higher ISS and MAIS, and higher preclinical mortality" T Stubig, M Petri, C Zeckey, S Brand, C Muller, D Otte, C Krettek C Haasper. November 2012 Alcohol Vol. 46, Issue 7, Pages 681-68
24. Blood or needle phobia as a defence under the Road Traffic Act 1988. K J B Rix Journal of clinical forensic medicine (1996) 3 173-177
25. Road Safety Research Report No 63 – Monitoring the Effectiveness of UK Field Impairment Tests, University of Glasgow, March 2006

26. A Review of Evidence Related to Drug Driving in the UK: A Report Submitted to the North Review Team. P.G Jackson and C J Hilditch, Clockwork Research Ltd. June 2010.
27. The relationship between the blood benzodiazepine concentration and performance in suspected impaired drivers. B E Smink, K J Lusthof, J J de Gier, D R A |uges, A C G Egberts. Journal of Forensic and Legal Medicine 15 (2008) 483-488.

Chapter 7 Just a scratch

28. The Edwin Smith Papyrus: the birth of analytical thinking in medicine and otolaryngology. <u>Stiefel M</u>, <u>Shaner A</u>, <u>Schaefer SD</u>. Laryngoscope. 2006 Feb;116(2):182-8.
29. Assessment of abuse-related injuries: A comparative study of forensic physicians, emergency room physicians, emergency room nurses and medical students. Udo JL, et al Journal of Forensic and Legal Medicine 15 (2008)15-19
30. The language of forensic medicine; the meaning of some terms employed. T Capper Medicine, Science and the Law (2001) vol 41 no 5.
31. Lack of agreement on colour descriptions between clinicians examinating childhood bruising. L A Munang, PA Leonard, JYQ Mok. Journal of Clinical Forensic Medicine (2002) 9 171-174.
32. Visual assessment of the timing of bruising by forensic experts. M I Pilling, P. Vanezis, D Perrett, A Johnson, Journal of Forensic and Legal Medicine. 17 (2010) 143-149

Chapter 8 The drug scene

33. Drugs of Dependence: the role of medical practitioners BMA

34. buzz.bournemouth.ac.uk/a-class-drugs-policy-timeline
35. The British National Formulary September 2013
36. Cawich S et al. Treating cocaine body packers: the unspoken personal risks. Journal of Forensic and Legal Medicine 2008; 15: 231-234.
37. Norfolk G. The fatal case of a cocaine body-stuffer and a literature review- towards evidence based management. Journal of Forensic and Legal Medicine 2007; 14: 49-52. 10.
38. Marc B. Managing high risk body-stuffers who swallow the evidence. Journal of Forensic and Legal Medicine 2008; 15: 200-201.
39. R J Booker, J E Smith, M P Rodger. "Packers, pushers and stuffers—managing patients with concealed drugs in UK emergency departments: a clinical and medicolegal review" *Emerg Med J* 2009;26:316-320
40. HM Government. Healthy lives, healthy people: our strategy for public health in England. 2010. www.gov.uk/government/uploads/system/uploads/attachment_data/file/136384/healthy_lives_healthy_people.pdf

Chapter 9 Problems with booze

41. HM Government. Government's alcohol strategy. 2012. www.gov.uk/government/uploads/system/uploads/attachment_data/file/224075/alcohol-strategy.pdf
42. Office for National Statistics. Alcohol related deaths in the United Kingdom, 2011. Stat Bull2013www.ons.gov.uk/ons/dcp171778_296289.pdf

Chapter 10 One for the pot

43. "On cannabis or Indian hemp" W Ley Read before the Royal Medico-Botanical Society. BMJ 1847

Chapter 11 Dowers from opium to valium

44. Opium as an international problem" The Geneva Conferences W.W Willoughby.

   a. Professor of Political Science at the Johns Hopkins University; The John Hopkins Press 1925

45. F. Aragon-Poce, E Martinez-Ferndez, C Marquez-Espinos, A Perez, R Mora, L.M. Torres. "History of Opium". International Congress Series 1242 (2002) 19-21
46. Ian Scott "Heroin: A Hundred-Year Habit" History Today Volume: 48 Issue: 6 1998
47. Giles M. 'Nutshells, criminal law' Published Sweet and Maxwell London 1996, Medicine Science and the Law (1998) Vol 38 No3 page 273
48. Ferner R.E. 'Forensic Pharmacology - Medicines, Mayhem and Malpractice' Published Oxford 1996 page 168-9
49. Cassidy M T, Curtis M, Muir G. Oliver J S "Drug abuse deaths in Glasgow in 1992 - a retrospective study". Medicine Science and the Law July 1995 Vol 35 No 3 page 207 - 212
50. Jamieson, R.J. "Methadone and heroin use: a survey of prisoners in Police Custody" Journal of Forensic and Legal Medicine 18 (2011) 233
51. National records for Scotland,"Drug related deaths in Scotland in 2011" www.gro-scotland.gov.uk.
52. Malcom Lader "A History of benzodiazepine dependence" *Journal of Substance Abuse Treatment*, Vol. 8, pp. *53-59, 1991*
53. The British National Formulary. February 2014
54. Symptoms and signs of substance misuse" Margaret Stark, Jason Payne-James. Pub Greenwich-medical. 2003.
55. "intheknowzone.com"

Chapter 12 Most haste less speed

56. Ailments through the ages. Richard Gordon Michael O'Mara books 1998
57. Pseudoephedrine and ephedrine: Managing the risk of misuse of medicines – July 2010 update MRHA
58. Review of deaths related to taking ecstasy, England and Wales, 1997-2000
(Published 11 January 2003) BMJ 2003;326:80
59. Acute excited states and sudden death; Much journalism, little evidence BMJ 1997;315:1107 Frank R Farnham, Henry G Kennedy,
60. Domhnall MacAuley ' Drugs in Sport' BMJ Vol 313 27th July 1996.
61. S.L. Elkin et al 'Bodybuilders find it easy to obtain insulin to help them in training' letter to B.M.J. Vol 314 26th April 1997
62. John Honour. 'Misuse of natural hormones in sport'. The Lancet Vol 349 21st June 1997.
63. Steven Karch "A History of Cocaine" published The Royal Society of Medicine 2003
64. Paul Vallely. "Drug that spans the Ages: The History of Cocaine." The Independent 2nd March 2006
65. Tony Wildsmith Chapter 1, "History and development of local anaesthesia" in "Principles and practice of regional anaesthesia 4th Ed" pub Oxford University Press 2012.
66. "People of the First Crusade" Michael Foss. Arcade Publishing; 1st edition (Oct 1997)

Chapter 13 Nothing but the truth

67. John Mortimer Presents 'The Trials of Marshall Hall' (Unabridged) by Michael Butt (16 Jan 2008)

68. Mozley and Whiteley ed E R Hardy Ivamy." Law Dictionary" 11th ed 1993 Butterworths
69. William Geldart "Introduction to English Law" Oxford University Press

Chapter 14 You're nicked, son

70. "The New Police Surgeon" ed S H Burges. Pub Hutchinson Benham 1978
71. "Miscellaneous Intelligence". Lond J Med 1850;0:505 (Published 03 May 1850)
72. Police and Criminal Evidence Act 1984 (PACE) Codes of Practice. 2011.
73. "Consent: patients and doctors making decisions together" published by General Medical Council 2008.
74. "Confidentiality" published by General Medical Council 2009
75. Website justice.org.uk
76. "A tiered healthcare system for persons in Police Custody – use of a forensic nursing service" S Young, D Wells G Jackson Journal of Clinical forensic Medicine (1994) 1 21-25
77. "Guidance on the safer detention and handling of persons in Police Custody" 2012 Pub ACPO NPIA

Chapter 15 Anything you say

78. "Fitness to be interviewed and the appropriate adult scheme: a survey of police surgeons' attitude". G A Norfolk. Journal of Clinical Forensic Medicine (1996) 3 (9-13)
79. "Fitness to interview during Police detention; a conceptual framework for forensic assessment" Gudjonsson, G Journal of Forensic Psychiatry. 1995, 6 1185-197

80. "Fitness to interview: current trends, views and an approach to the assessment procedure" J A Gall & I Freckelton. Journal of clinical forensic medicine. (1999) 6 213-223.
81. "Fitness to interview during Police detention; a conceptual framework for forensic assessment" Gudjonsson, G Journal of Forensic Psychiatry. 1995, 6 1185-197
82. "Persons at risk during interviews in police custody: identification of vulnerabilities" Gudjonsson et al Research study 12 Royal Commission on criminal justice London HMSO 1993

Chapter 16 Born evil?

83. Journal of investigative psychology and offender profiling 1:1-15 (2004)
84. The Anatomy of violence. Adrian Raine pub Allen Lane 2013
85. Child care and the growth of love. John Bowbly. 1953 pub Penguin Books
86. NICE guidance CG77 Antisocial personality disorder: Treatment, management and prevention. Issued Jan 2009, modified Sept 2013.

Chapter 17 All Change

91 Elias, Norbert. *The Civilizing Process.* Vols. 1–2. Oxford: Oxford University 1978

Printed in Great Britain
by Amazon